Old Age: The Last Segregation

This book is printed on one hundred per cent recycled paper.

In the same series:

*Ralph Nader's
Study Group Report
on Nursing Homes*

OLD AGE
The Last Segregation

Claire Townsend, PROJECT DIRECTOR

Grossman Publishers
New York   1971

THE TASK FORCE

CLAIRE TOWNSEND, Task Force Director
   Graduate, 1970, Miss Porter's School, Farmington,
   Connecticut; Freshman, Princeton University
KATE BLACKWELL, Editor
   B.A., Wellesley College; M.A., University of North
   Carolina
RALPH NADER, Special Consultant
ELIZABETH BALDWIN
   Graduate, 1970, Miss Porter's School
JANET KEYES
   Graduate, 1970, Miss Porter's School; Freshman, Mt.
   Holyoke College
LALLIE LLOYD
   Graduate, 1970, Miss Porter's School; Freshman,
   Princeton University
CATHERINE MORGAN
   Graduate, 1970, Miss Porter's School; Freshman,
   Boston University
PATRICIA PITTIS
   Graduate, 1970, Miss Porter's School; Freshman, St.
   John's College at Annapolis
MARGARET QUINN
   B.A., Randolph-Macon Woman's College; Instructor,
   Miss Porter's School
Andrea Hricko, Research Assistant
   B.A., Connecticut College; M.P.H., University of
   North Carolina
Susan Fagin, Production Director
   B.A., Olivet College

INTRODUCTION BY RALPH NADER

Twenty million Americans—10 per cent of the population—are over sixty-five years old. Within a hyperbolic youth-oriented society and economy, these citizens are being increasingly "structured" out of their just share of material, psychological, and social benefits. "Out of sight, out of mind" is perhaps the most succinct description of the workings of institutional and individual forces on the elderly. More and more they are separated from the rest of society, by a kind of geriatric segregation as consumers, residents, relatives, victims, and other roles which they choose or are compelled to assume.

The statistical profile of the over-sixty-five Americans displays an aggregation of poverty, sickness, loneliness, powerlessness. In one routine category of standard of living after another, they register far below the average and often compare with the deprived or oppressed status of minority groups. The conventional injustices of the land bear down heavily on the elderly. Consumer fraud, inflation, fixed pensions and social security benefits, street crime, absence of mass transit, spiraling rents and housing costs, swelling medical and drug bills, and the virtual end of the extended family unit have a severe discriminatory impact on old people. The recent Senate report, *Developments in Aging, 1969,* provides such dismaying data in compelling fashion. But most gnawing and omnipresent is the psychological devastation heaped on the old by a society that lets them know in many ways, small and large, that they are no longer wanted, no longer useful, no longer filled with life's potential and warmth—in short, that they're considered a drag.

There is a colossal amount of collective callousness that pervades society, from the organization to the individual levels. The most intense focus of what has been wrought for old people is the nursing home. The few homes that are humane, competent, and mindful of their residents' need for activity and meaning in their day highlight the staggering gap between what an affluent society should attain and what is too frequently the reality for most nursing homes.

The full scope of nursing home abuses and profiteering has yet to be told. Although the Federal government pours over a billion dollars a year into this two-and-a-half billion dollar industry through Medicare and other subsidy programs, there have neither been the full-fledged Congressional hearings, nor the enforcement of adequate Federal and state standards, nor the administrative inquiries and disclosures that are needed to reduce the institutional violence and cruelty that are rampant. Such moves have not occurred in spite of major fire disasters, fatal food contaminations, corporate manipulations, drug experimentation beyond proper medical discretion, kickbacks in drug sales for the residents, abysmal lack of medical supervision, and strong evidence that such abuses are more epidemic than episodic.

Early in 1970, six seniors and a young instructor at Miss Porter's School in Farmington, Connecticut, responded enthusiastically to the suggestion that they constitute a task force to study nursing home conditions and the responsibilities of the Federal government therein. Starting work in the spring, they saw the heart-rending tragedies firsthand. During the summer their work ranged from working experience inside several nursing homes to intensive study of documents and complaints, and interviewing officials.

What follows is their contribution, as young citizens reaching out to old citizens, coupled with their determination that something concrete be done by those in authority to comfort the afflicted. How quickly such action will commence can be significantly affected by the needed emergence of a retired people's "liberation movement" focusing on the economic, governmental, and social injustices heaped upon them because they have grown old. Abundant experience, time, and organizational talent can be mustered, once the clarion call resounds through the land that retired people will no longer be phased out, manipulated, herded, patronized, and rendered futile by a society insensitive to the diverse rights and potential contributions of older people.

Nursing homes are only one facet of the overall subculture for the aged that is being created without their participation and because of their powerlessness. It is time for these retired people to become involved citizens for their own sake and for those who come after them.

December, 1970
Washington, D.C.

A MODEST PROPOSAL

They wander aimlessly down busy sidewalks, so the rest of us push them aside. Bus and train stations are crowded with them, though they rarely buy tickets. They huddle in doorways in full view of the public. They are America's aged. They number twenty million. Most of them, fortunately, are invisible most of the time. Only one million are permanently invisible, in institutions; others are afraid or unable to leave the rooms where they live. But the ones who do venture into the streets are an unpleasant reminder of a serious national problem.

Since they are forced to retire at sixty-five, and since only a few have enough money to live on, most of the aged depend upon their families or the state for their welfare. Everyone agrees that this situation is not satisfactory. Most families cannot keep their old parents at home because of social and economic pressure, and many old parents will not accept public assistance because of pride or ignorance. If they do accept funds from the state, they are barely able to eke out an existence on their meager allotments. At least one-third are forced to spend the remaining years of their lives alone or with strangers, of no use to society or to themselves.

If they live with their families, it is under strained conditions. If they live alone, or with an equally old and disabled friend, they find climbing flights of stairs to an unheated one-room apartment tiring and discouraging. They are afraid to leave their apartments in any case, fully aware that, weakened and defenseless, they are choice targets for street crime. Money is their major problem, though most were not poor until they became old.

They do not fit into society, they are not wanted in society; they themselves just want to die or be cared for until they do die.

One of the nation's growing concerns is the population explosion. All the clamor so far has been about birth control—but why cut down on the number of children? They are fun to have around! Why not cut down instead on the increasing number of old people, who are *not* fun to have around, who merely clutter our streets, break our backs financially, are an eyesore, and a drag on our economic growth? Which would we rather have around —a lot of bright young faces filled with energy and enthusiasm, or a crowd of wrinkled old faces filled with loneliness and despair?

Look at the problem another way. You love your dog, but he is old now and you have sadly watched as his health deteriorates. The money you have spent to keep him alive is of no use; he continues to grow older and sicker, becomes more and more arthritic, loses both weight and hair. He cannot eat any more, and all he does is whine mournfully. You cannot bear to see him in this painful condition—after all, we are an humane society—and you cannot bear to see this ugly parody of the playful, beautiful puppy he used to be. And so you put him to sleep.

To treat the aged similarly would be inhumane, but there is another scheme that should work just as well. In fact, the government has actually been perpetuating the idea for some time. The government's unquestioning support of the nursing home industry has helped keep the aged away from society.

The nursing home alternative is presently very expensive, but the cost may be considered relatively low when the benefits are taken into account, and few live for long in a nursing home anyway. Patient neglect and generally poor treatment are already widespread and the public need only continue to do nothing for conditions to worsen.

Consider the following: the more bedridden patients there are in a home, the better for the institution (less work, more government money). Patients may therefore simply be tied down in beds and wheelchairs until they lose the use of their legs. Bedsores are easy to incur if the beds are left wet or if no sheet is placed between the patient and the rubber mat. Sedatives can be freely prescribed to keep the patients gentle and quiet. The emergency call button can be placed out of reach, or the signal can simply be ignored. The meal trays, too, can be placed out of reach. Water may be refused, or doled out in tiny disposable medicine cups, which can be reused later. If the patients are fed, the food may be the refuse of a restaurant or hotel, or damaged goods from the supermarket. Food poisoning is another effective kill-all. The food may be served tasteless, cold, and in insufficient amounts, so patients die from malnutrition or dehydration. Even an overdose of laxatives will do the trick, or a gradually increasing dose of the wrong medicine. Mentally disturbed patients, moved in at the convenience of state mental institutions, may end up injuring their roommates or themselves. Patients can also be burned to death because of accidents from smoking in bed, or because they are unable to turn off the hot water in the shower, or turn down the electric blanket in bed. Patients can be frozen to death if wheeled outside in thirty-degree weather wearing very little clothing, or if left in front of an open window at night without sheets or nightclothes, or perhaps if the air conditioning is too cold.

The advantages are clear: a decline in the population, fewer mouths to feed, fewer people to worry about and take care of, more money for the deprived children of our nation, more money for education and schools, and, on the whole, a younger, more attractive population. The beauty of the plan is that it may be executed out of sight of the public. It may even be worth considering a compulsory age for entrance into a nursing home, shall we say seventy?

The proposal is not as modest as it may seem. The incidents cited here have actually occurred, are occurring now, in nursing homes across the nation. This report attempts to document the crisis in American nursing home care, to discover, if possible, what has gone wrong, and to recommend improvements and changes.

Early in the project of summer, 1970, we became convinced that a study of nursing homes must necessarily be broad-based. An overview of nursing homes must deal with current efforts of the Federal government to regulate important aspects of a privately controlled industry. The modern nursing home must be understood in a context of past attempts to provide health care for the elderly through legislation. The economic and social conditions of the elderly outside the nursing home must be considered. Finally, society's attitude toward the elderly is a crucial factor in understanding why nursing homes are so often places of pain and despair rather than comfort and hope.

We attempted to cover many areas of care for the elderly in order to trace the reasons for conditions in nursing homes and to suggest alternatives for improvement. Members of the team took specific areas of responsibility for this task: Claire Townsend and Patricia Pittis investigated government involvement in nursing homes. Catherine Morgan was responsible for analyzing legislation affecting the elderly. Lallie Lloyd studied financial aspects of the nursing home. Janet Keyes studied personnel, health care, and overall environment of the nursing home. Margaret Quinn made a detailed study of drugs used in nursing homes. Elizabeth Baldwin was concerned with the social and economic conditions of the elderly outside the nursing home.

In addition, all members of the team took part in a basic study of nursing homes as an institution.

This report is based on interviews with more than eighty-five officials in the Federal government, state agencies, the nursing home industry, and the medical profession, all of whom are responsible for health care for the elderly. We utilized government reports and documents on care for the aged, and more than one hundred detailed letters and follow-ups received during the course of our investigation. This report also incorporates our observations and interviews while working in three nursing homes in the Washington area and visiting more than twenty nursing homes in Washington, Northern Virginia, Maryland, Connecticut, New York, and New Jersey.

The team wishes to acknowledge the cooperation of the many people who freely gave their time and shared their knowledge with us. Patricia Roberts, who until recently worked in Congressman David Pryor's office, was especially helpful. We are convinced that there are many individuals who care deeply about the elderly, who are trying to improve their position, and who are frustrated by the lack of support and resources for the task.

We are indebted to Kate Blackwell for her help in editing this report; to Andrea Hricko for her research assistance; and to Susan Fagin for production of the final result.

Our report does not attempt to be a professional critique of overall nursing home care, although it does include studies by professionals. We have been attacked because we are not professionals, but this is not a strong argument. Our nonprofessionalism may be in some respects a weakness, but in more important ways it is a strength. We have no vested interests to serve, no reason to keep silent about what we see, no cause to dole out praise or blame, no excuses to make on behalf of anyone or anything. Although we do not have the depth and length of professional experience, we have acquired a breadth of knowledge about the nursing home and the problems of aging in American society. We hope that we, unlike some of the professionals we interviewed and occasionally criticized in our report, can see the forest despite the trees. Our youth and the necessary brevity of our study are not valid arguments against what we say here. If we have been too harsh, we are pleased that the aged are getting better treatment than what we saw; if, as seems more likely, we have been too gentle, we call upon those who are professionals to face the severity of the problems as professionals ought to.

We offer some examples of what occurs in nursing

homes across the country and an assessment of the problems based on our concern, as Americans who are not yet old, for the welfare and well-being of older citizens.

December, 1970   Elizabeth Baldwin
Washington, D.C.   Janet Keyes
                                  Lallie Lloyd
                                  Catherine Morgan
                                  Patricia Pittis
                                  Margaret Quinn
                                  Claire Townsend

CONTENTS

Old Age: The Last Segregation

1 *Introduction*

July 10, 1970

Dear Mr. Nader,

On July 7, our local newspaper carried an account of your latest project, an extensive inquiry into nursing homes. I cannot tell you how glad I am that you, and the group of researchers you have chosen, are conducting such an investigation. I only regret that I cannot join with you, personally. However, I feel so strongly about the need for such an investigation that I am compelled to write now and tell you briefly (if that is possible!) of my own experiences. . . .

One year ago, my parents, aged seventy-four and seventy-three, had a one-car accident in late afternoon on a rural country road in central Wisconsin. My father, who was driving, suffered what later was diagnosed as similar to an epileptic seizure—he was awake and aware, but totally immobilized for about thirty seconds—and the car careened across the road and into a farm driveway embankment. My father hit the rearview mirror and was knocked unconscious on impact. My mother, however, was thrown against the dash and suffered a compression fracture of her spine, leaving her instantly paralyzed from the waist down, although completely conscious.

My parents had been farmers all their married life,

and had successfully raised eight children—of whom I am the sixth. Despite a twenty-year span between oldest and youngest, our family has always been a very close one, even though we now are scattered throughout the United States. A month to the day before the accident, all eight children had been back to the farm for a five-day reunion. At the time of the accident, only two of us, a sister and myself, lived in our home state.

My father's only injury was a severe gash over his left eye. However, a milogram performed on my mother showed an obstruction in her spinal column, and the family doctor had her transferred on June 17 to a hospital in Milwaukee, to be put under the care of Dr. B., a neurosurgeon. He operated on June 18, removed a bone chip that was pressing on her spinal cord, and told us that in all probability she would remain paralyzed the rest of her life, although he admitted there was no sure way of knowing. Any recovery she might have would be spontaneous, and the most that could be done for her would be physical therapy designed to keep her muscles from atrophying and to keep her joints limber. * * * hospital is extremely well equipped for such therapy and my mother began it within a week of her surgery.

The accident meant the end of my parents' life on the farm. My father had been slowly growing senile in the past two years, and my mother, the strong, hard-working wife, had kept his growing memory loss, his general ineptness cloaked as much as she could. She filled in the gaps in his competency so well that even we children, who could see his mental deterioration, had no idea of the extremity of it until she was hospitalized and we found Daddy literally could not function without her. I stayed with my father at the farm until Mama was transferred by ambulance to Milwaukee on the 17th, and then my father moved into my house with me for three weeks. . . . It was a peculiarly hard time; my husband had decided only the week before the accident to change jobs and move to Indiana in August, for two years. Our house in Milwaukee had to be rented out for the duration.

We had suddenly a hundred imperative decisions to make about our parents. My father had sunk almost immediately into a deep depression; he, the strong, dominating father whom we never had seen cry, wept uncontrollably day and night. He had lucid spells, of course, in which he seemed almost the same hard, thoughtful, and clear-thinking man he had always been. But his grief and guilt over Mama's paralysis were truly agony. Mama and the farm were all he had lived for, really, and now he had nothing to live for any more. We eight kids discussed and planned endlessly. Mama had three months of Medicare coverage while in * * * hospital, which set her discharge date at September 17. If Daddy could only come out of his depression enough to try to look ahead to a new life with her, even confined to a wheelchair, we thought it was still possible that they might be able to live in town, in a community with helpful friends and neighbors. With that in mind, two of my sisters hunted around in a small town nearby the farm and found a small house in a beautiful location within the folks' financial means.

All that long summer, the one thing that kept my mother's spirits up was the thought that she might still be able to live a nearly normal life, and buying that house was the best thing possible for her morale. We had discussed it with Dr. B. beforehand, and he had agreed that it was a very sensible idea—not only the house, but the fact that it was in the only town in the area (within a sixty- or seventy-mile radius) that also had a physical therapy clinic. He referred all his patients within that area to the local doctor who ran the clinic, he told us, and assured us that the therapy there was excellent, and the doctor very good.

The physical therapy clinic, we discovered, was located within a nursing home. Dr. M., the doctor in charge, worked in another building . . . but also owned the nursing home, which is run by a Mr. F., and outpatients as well as patients used the physical therapy facilities. My sisters inspected the nursing home, which seemed very clean and well run, talked at length with both Dr. M. and Mr. F., and came away satisfied with the facilities.

In the meantime my father continued to grow worse. He refused to eat, and his depression grew more and more severe. We took him to see a psychiatrist who recommended that he be hospitalized in a psychiatric ward. During the week he was there, routine physical tests revealed an unidentifiable spot on his lung. He was then transferred into the care of a Dr. L., who, on September 11, performed surgery, removing one-fourth of his right lung. The cause of the spot was never diagnosed—or, if it was, never revealed to us.

On September 17, 1969, Dr. B. transferred my mother to * * * nursing home, under the care of Dr. M. He told my sister that under the circumstances it was impossible for my mother to live alone in the house; since my father was physically incapable of caring for her, the best solution at the moment was for her to be admitted directly to the nursing home where she would get continuing therapy and care.

During the summer the entire family was kept informed of every single development concerning our parents. I wrote a weekly newsletter (Xeroxing seven copies) and mailed it out until I moved, and my sister continued the practice. Our telephone bills never averaged less than thirty dollars per month—the eight of us discussed plans endlessly. We visited our mother twice a day every day, while she was in * * * hospital, and I had endless talks with the social workers, the doctor (when he deigned to talk with us), and followed Mama through her daily routine in therapy. We knew exactly what she could do for herself, and what further things she could expect to accomplish. Never, at any time, did we ever expect that her full, useful life was ended. She was always in excellent physical condition, had worked hard all her life; her mind was clear and bright, and her correspondence alone while in the hospital showed how unusually well-liked a woman she is. Friends, relatives, and farm neighbors drove to Milwaukee regularly all summer to visit her. We told Dr. B. all that (most of it he was aware of, anyway), and when he suggested (decided, rather) that she go into the nursing home, we agreed with the understanding that it was a temporary solution until such time as further therapy would enable her to live in a home of her own again.

As my sister remarked in one of her newsletters that fall: ". . . I guess basically I do have confidence and trust in the honesty and capability of all these surgeons, specialists and the rest of the medical profession into whose hands the folks' lives have been thrust this summer, but that's only because if I did anything other than put trust in them I'd be a nervous wreck. They certainly wield a lot of power over the directions of peoples' lives. . . ."

That's not a small point, Mr. Nader. People are at the mercy of their doctors' judgment. Particularly at a traumatic time. . . .

Our father continued to grow worse mentally, although he, like Mama, still had a body with the strength of an ox. . . . Ten days after his lung surgery he sat upright in the car and drove with my sister and her husband one hundred miles to the nursing home to be admitted as a patient with Mama, in a double room. He wanted desperately to be with her, and being with her seemed the only good thing we as a family could do for him at that point.

Other imperative matters needed attention; grain stored in the bins on the farm had to be hauled to town and sold that summer. My brother took care of that—coming from Virginia to do it. Hay had to be cut and baled—a neighbor offered to take care of that. And by fall we knew the folks would have to hold a farm auction to sell the machinery and farm equipment, and the household items that Mama would never use again. I spent a week at the farm in October, and with the help of the neighbors emptied the house of forty years of love and family living. My mother, in the nursing home, advised me which things she wanted sold, and which she wanted kept. I visited my parents there every night. My father no longer remembered that I had moved to Indiana, and had become very paranoic. He hallucinated regularly—most often at night—and his physical condition had deteriorated noticeably. He had lost so much weight his clothes hung on him. The auction was held

October 11; both my parents came to the farm for the entire day—my mother in her wheelchair, and my father with his ribs taped—he had fallen in the bathroom the night before and broken two ribs. But the auction was extremely successful, and the folks made enough money to take care of their medical bills—at least for a while.

I would like to skip over the next three months entirely, the memory is still so awful. I corresponded with my mother weekly; my father grew progressively worse, he hallucinated nights, got out of bed and crawled to my mother's bed and shook the rails, screaming out the nightmares he was living through. Nurses would rush in after Mama turned on her light, and with the help of a male aide would give my father a hypo and shove him back into bed. My mother, during this time, began to suffer increasing pain in her legs and lower back— nerve rejuvenation, the doctor called it—and did in fact regain slight movement in her right leg. Her nights were painful, and the little rest she was able to get was continually interrupted by my father. During the day they were left alone, and my mother had to watch my father constantly, ready to call for the nurses should he try to get out of bed or out of his chair and maneuver around. He was too weak to walk unaided. In short, for nine hundred dollars per month, plus medical care(!), my paralyzed mother was given the job of caring for my father twenty-four hours a day. Dr. M. never came to see either of them.

Shortly after Thanksgiving my sister and her husband drove to the nursing home to see Dr. M. (a special trip, on Friday—they came every weekend to see the folks, but Dr. M. honored his Sabbath on Saturday, and was thus unavailable to them). They were very concerned about Daddy's health. He had lost so much weight his dentures no longer fitted, and he could not eat what food he was inclined to eat. They asked about what medication he was getting; since his discharge after lung surgery he had been given innumerable pills daily, along with the dilantin prescribed in June to control the epileptic-type seizures. His vision was bad—he complained of seeing double most of the time—and of course he had lost his sense of balance. Dr. M. smiled sweetly at my sister and assured her that he would see about re-fitting the dentures, and would check over the medication, although it was all antibiotics, given to curb any infection that might arise from the September surgery, he said.

In the meantime, both another sister in California and I had become terribly upset because Mama's letters indicated she was getting little if any rest at all during the nights. Both of us wrote to Dr. M. I wrote requesting that my father be moved across the hall into a separate room to insure that Mama would get some rest at night, and my sister wrote suggesting that Daddy might be better cared for at this point in the state mental hospital. We both wrote asking for advice, and asking that we get replies.

Neither of us received any acknowledgment of our letters. But on December 7, 1969, two nurses and a male aide rushed into my parents' room at the nursing home and forcibly removed my father into a waiting ambulance, in which he was transferred to the state hospital. My mother was frantic, and begged to know why. After a good while, Dr. M. came to see her and told her that Daddy had been transferred there at the request of two of her daughters. Since Daddy had grown uncontrollable and unsubduable, he judged it the best course of action. My mother telephoned my sister in Milwaukee to tell her the news. My sister was, understandably, terribly upset and extremely angry with both me and my sister in California. She phoned Dr. M. and he told her that we had both written to him and demanded that our father be put there.

I happen to be very careful about keeping copies of all my pertinent correspondence; I had only requested that Daddy be moved to a separate room, and had said, ". . . I want to make it clear that I am only one of eight children—certainly my decision alone shouldn't be the final one. . . ." I had asked for, and expected to receive, advice from the doctor.

Perhaps I need not even add that my father never had his medication checked or altered by Dr. M., nor were his dentures refitted.

On January 20, 1970, my father died in the state hospital. He had starved himself into a living skeleton. . . . At Christmas he did not recognize my sister nor my brother when they came to see him. . . . In his dreams he was still whole and farming, and kept trying to get up and leave, saying that it was such a long, cold spring, and he had to get back to the farm to get the crops in. . . .

My father wanted to die, I know; I do not mean to make it sound as though he was neglected totally—he had willed himself to die. But his transfer from the nursing home to the state hospital was done cruelly and unnecessarily, with absolutely no thought for my mother, or for any of his children—let alone him.

And that left my mother. In January, I drove again to Wisconsin and saw her and talked at length with the therapist in charge of her, a very nice, personable young man. He told me that what Mama needed, now that Daddy was gone, was to get into * * * Rehabilitation Institute in Milwaukee. There was much she could learn to do for herself from a wheelchair, and she just was not learning to do it at the nursing home. "She's spoiled here," he said, "she's the only patient here who has a clear mind and the nurses all visit with her and do everything for her—they won't let her do anything for herself. . . ."

Can you get her there right away, I asked. I can't do it, he said apologetically. Dr. M. has to sign the order . . . I'm only the therapist. . . .

Mama had changed; her indomitable spirit, which shone through everything all that summer at the hospital, was gone. Everywhere nurses cluck-clucked over her; her catheter was well in evidence on her wheelchair, and she complained that her back brace (fitted on her directly after surgery) was never put on properly. She showed us the weals to prove it. I gave her a long Dutch-uncle talk about doing more for herself; when she had come to the nursing home from the hospital, she had been able to transfer from bed to wheelchair all alone. At the nursing home they had put her sliding board away in a closet and chose instead to use two nurses to get her in and out of bed. Still, I told her, she must learn to be more self-sufficient in order to live anywhere else, and I told her she must plan on going to the rehabilitation institute.

From January to April the family postponed getting Mama into the Institute because Mama had decided that Daddy's memorial service (he had donated his body to the state university medical school) should be held in the spring, his favorite time of year. She had asked that all eight kids cooperate in writing and planning the entire service. We did, and in April all eight of us again came home. The service was beautifully put together and conducted by all of us, in the Unitarian church on April 19.

However, on Friday, April 17, my sister from California and I drove to see Dr. M. We asked him to admit Mama to the rehabilitation institute at once, and told him again of our hopes for her future. He stood in his office and laughed at us. He told us that our mother was an incurable invalid, that she could never expect to live outside an institution, and he hooted at me: "Why, do you realize it takes three nurses just to get her in and out of bed?" I asked him why, since she had come there from the hospital able to do it all by herself, and he changed the subject. He cited her back brace, her catheter, her constant night pain, all as irrefutable evidence that she would never be able to leave that nursing home.

And we looked at his flabby, vacuous face and saw that he looked at our mother and knew only a seventy-four-year-old farm woman who owned a 120-acre farm, thirty acres of good lake-shore property with cabin, and a value-increasing house in his town, not half a block away from his own house. He owned a nursing home filled with patients, and of all of them, our mother was the most secure financial liability he had, I know. He could keep her there until she died and own everything she had. . . .

If Mama had had good nursing care there all that while, we would not have been so boiling mad, but we knew from her letters and from my sister's newsletters what kind of care she had been given. When she complained about her night pain, the doctor told her to take an extra pill (we were never told what she was being given), but the nurses would not give it to her because the doctor had not bothered to put it on her chart. Daytime she was in constant pain from the back brace because the nurses could not be bothered to take the time to put it on properly; it kept pressing into and opening a bedsore she had incurred almost a year before. When she complained of pain in her bladder, the nurses told her she was imagining things. When they rolled her over to change her bed sheets, urine spilled out all over; her catheter, newly inserted the day before, had been put in improperly, and had not been draining. . . . They charged her for the new one they had to put in. The doctor never came to see her more than once a month, and then stood in the doorway and asked how she felt—never examined her at all. And if he saw her in the hall on her way to the dining room, he charged her for a visit; I know, I have seen the bills. He refused to submit any of her initial bills to Medicare, saying they would not pay them anyway. When the local banker (who was appointed executor when Daddy died) and the lawyer who works with him came to see Mr. F., the administrator, about the bills, they were kept waiting for one hour by the receptionist, and then told that Mr. F. was unable to see them that day. And a few days later, Dr. M. came in to see my mother and told her that unless she paid up her bill in full immediately, she would not go anywhere, let alone to the rehabilitation institute.

To go into more detail, I would have to cite the long visit I had this month with the banker, the executor of Daddy's estate. He saw Mama regularly all those months, and knows the harassment, both mental and physical, she got at the nursing home.

Last winter my home-town newspaper did a series of articles on nursing homes. The tone of those articles was how awful it was the way families subject their elderly members to such places. That may be true in some cases but not always, and the villains who are so carefully never exposed are most of the time those grand, outstanding members of the medical profession at whose mercy the public is. . . .

In our visit with Dr. M., he told my sister and me

that he had "no objection" to my mother being admitted to the rehabilitation institute, but that he thought the person to admit her was her surgeon of the summer before, Dr. B. And, he added, Dr. B. was coming to the local hospital the following Tuesday. Perhaps he would drive out and see our mother then, and make the arrangements.

Neither my sister nor I trusted Dr. M., so when we drove back to Milwaukee that night I phoned Dr. B. I told him of our visit with Dr. M. and what he had said. He was very cold and unconcerned, but finally agreed to see my mother, providing she could get herself to the hospital no later than 10:15 A.M. on Tuesday morning. After the memorial service for my father on Sunday, I arranged with friends of my mother to drive her there Tuesday.

Dr. B. kept her waiting for one hour. She was there by 10:00 A.M. I suspect that he spent a large portion of the time on the telephone with Dr. M., since my mother saw him coming out of surgery and walking down the hall more than half an hour before he bothered to see her. He began the visit by telling her coldly and bluntly that she would never walk again. Then, when she asked him about getting her into the Institute for an evaluation at least, he said yes, he would do that. Period.

Two days later my sister in Milwaukee telephoned him and asked him when he would have Mama admitted. He told her, in an extremely nasty way, that he was not her doctor, would never again be her doctor; since Dr. M. *was* her physician, he was the only one able to admit her to the Institute for any reason.

At that my sister wisely telephoned the Institute. They in turn called both doctors, and the upshot was that my mother was transferred there on May 31, 1970. I took the train to Milwaukee that night, and spent the entire following day there with my mother and the doctors, nurses, therapists, and social worker.

My talk with the social worker was very illuminating. I told her of the letters a sister and I had written to both Drs. B. and M., after the visit to Wisconsin in April, requesting that they admit our mother. She told me what both surely knew—that Mama had never needed more than a member of the family's or her own request to be transferred. In the end, it was Dr. B. not Dr. M. who had signed the admitting papers, but my sister could have done it equally well.

And now, after only five weeks at the Institute, my mother has proven what we in the family knew all along —that she is more than capable of taking care of herself, with only minimal supervision. The back brace was taken away at once; she had not needed it for six months, the doctor told me. She irrigates her own catheter, controls her own bowel program, can wash and dress herself, and get in and out of bed without help. Her pain is due to muscle spasms; the medication prescribed by Dr. M. was diagnosed as a strong narcotic, which was discarded the first night at the Institute. In its place she has a muscle relaxant and a sleeping pill, and is sleeping soundly for the first time in nine months. She is using a sewing machine again, can work a rug loom, can roll over, turn herself, pull and drag herself anywhere on a mat or floor, and can do fifteen push-ups without getting even short of breath. She can work in a kitchen, do her own laundry and ironing and, in short, is as self-sufficient as any person can be without the full use of her legs.

She will be discharged from the Institute the first week in August and, I am happy to say, will then move in here with me. She is great, just great—I cannot tell you how much I am looking forward to having her here, nor how pleased my husband and kids are.

Far from the futile picture that charlatan owning the nursing home painted, she has a bright and full life ahead of her. She comes from a long-lived family—her father died at ninety-five, still articulate and clear of mind—and all eight kids are looking forward to long visits from her throughout the years. She loved to travel, and the last few years she and Daddy visited Texas every winter. Dr. P., her doctor at the Institute, assured her and me that she can still travel, by airplane, and enjoy her visits as much as she ever did.

But the best part of all is seeing Mama once again feeling useful and self-confident. If she had had to stay in that nursing home, she would have died. That is not just my opinion; the social worker told me the psychologist had confirmed it after all her tests at the Institute. The nursing home staff treated her as a total invalid and expected her to waste away and die. Far from caring about her future as a whole human being, that bastard of a doctor did his utmost to convince her children as well as her that her life was over. A caring family was the last thing he wanted for one of his patients.

I am convinced that my case is certainly not an exception. It is not only the nursing homes and the appalling care they give patients who need to be investigated, it is the doctors who own and live off them, and the cohorts who transfer patients to them.

The entire medical profession has one hell of a lot of answering to do for their treatment of elderly people. From the glib practitioners who recommend nursing homes as the only solution to distraught families to the money suckers who bleed the life's work of old people and call it "care." My mother earned every cent of her money, and by God, we eight kids intend to see to it that she spends it all on herself, enjoying herself to the fullest until she dies. She is lucky; her bills are in the thousands of dollars, but she has the money to pay them all and still live comfortably and well. What about all the old people who have only their homes when tragedy such as this strikes? I have learned a lot about such cases in the past year, believe me. I know about nursing homes that have their patients sign over all their property in return for "care" until they die. And I know about the homes themselves—the one my mother existed in for nine months, for example. She had a TV in her room, and every day all the nurses piled in to watch their favorite soap operas. She bought a paper every night, and during the night the nurses stole in and lifted it off her bed, thinking she was asleep; and she never got to finish reading it. . . . I could go on and on. . . . They took advantage of her clear mind and her money-paying ability, and treated her like a rotten vegetable ready to be discarded.

I am mad. Not only for my mother, for I know she is never going back to one of those places, but for all the people who have still to endure those nursing homes; the ones who cannot cry out for help themselves, and

who have no families to do it for them—and who else
is there to care?

EXCERPT FROM A JOURNAL *

July 10, 1970

At 2:45, fifteen minutes before I was to go off duty,
the head nurse caught me in the lobby of the residence
where I was temporarily working, and told me to go
outside to watch a certain old lady (whom I will call
Mrs. Smith). I was to keep her at the main entrance,
because her sister was coming to pick her up to take
her back to their nearby apartment.

By the time I was outside the front door, Mrs. Smith
was at the end of the next block, trotting at full speed.
I caught up with her and asked where she was going
at such a speed, and why she was leaving when she
knew that her sister would be expecting her in a short
while at the front entrance. Mrs. Smith said she knew
how to get to her sister's apartment. Not wanting to
cause her sister extra trouble, she was going to walk to
the apartment herself. I told Mrs. Smith that she would
be creating more complications if she started walking
toward the apartment and missed her sister.

This did not deter her. She crossed the street and
started down the next block. Until I could think of a
more convincing argument, I had no hope of keeping
her near the home. I told her there was a prospect of a
rainstorm coming up. She simply stated that her coat
was lined and could stand a little rain—and she walked
on unabashed.

At this point, I had three alternatives: to run back
to the home, get help, and hope to find her again; to try
to walk her back to the home by force; or to walk
with her to her sister's apartment. I chose to try to
walk her back by force, but found this to be fruitless,
since she was at least as strong as I was, if not stronger.
We began walking again, with her leading the way,

* This report quotes frequently from journals kept by members
of the study group while working in nursing homes. The following section is from Patricia Pittis' journal.

but soon I realized that she had no idea where her sister's apartment was located. Although she claimed she was going to a meeting of a group she belonged to, it was evident that she was simply wandering about aimlessly. I began to worry because I did not know how long this would last, nor where she would take me.

After we had walked at least six blocks away from the home, I stopped to call the head nurse. I gave her our whereabouts, asked her what I should do, and would she please send someone stronger or more persuasive to bring Mrs. Smith back to the home, because I just could not prevent her from going wherever she pleased.

The head nurse answered, "Don't leave her; keep walking with her."

"But what about picking us up? Will you send someone to get us?"

"We'll see what we can do," she answered.

Mrs. Smith and I walked on and on—and no help arrived. I was beginning to feel quite absurd and ignorant of the next best step to take. By this time, it was at least 3:30 P.M. It was also obvious that no one was straining himself to find us, although it would have been almost impossible in such a maze of city streets. I hailed a cab, but when the driver finally stopped at the end of the next block and saw how much trouble I was having trying to coax Mrs. Smith toward the taxi, the cabbie impatiently drove away.

By now I was worried, frustrated, tired, and unable to handle this old woman, who was nearing her eighties. No one in the home had bothered to give me even a short briefing on her mental health and stability before she was placed totally in my custody. Her conversation was sporadic, nonsequential, and often unintelligible; and yet, I was still unsure as to whether her memory was failing, or how much of what she was saying was worth believing, and if not, then how to interpret her speech. Maybe she was perfectly sane, and was putting on an act so I would leave her alone. I did not know— no doctor or nurse had told me anything about her condition, and, having started work at the home only three days before, I had no experience to guide me.

With the help of a young man, I hailed a police car.

The young man's wife called the home again to tell them where we were, and to please come pick us up. We must have stood at the end of that block for fifteen minutes, trying to persuade Mrs. Smith to get into the police car with me. There was still no sign of anyone from the home to help us out. They had no excuse this time for they had the address and should have already appeared. Two policemen tried to carry Mrs. Smith into the car. She kicked and shouted, "I am a grown woman, and I will never think highly of the police again after this!" The police tried to bribe her by taking her hat and saying they would not give it back until she got in the car, but no amount of argument would entice her.

It did not take more than a few minutes before all the neighborhood windows and doors were filled with curious spectators, children were crowding around asking me what Mrs. Smith had done, and a public bus had taken the opportunity to stop and watch the spectacle. All that was missing was a reporter and a TV camera. No one knew what to do; the police were embarrassed, a woman was shouting at me that Mrs. Smith was perfectly sane and had the right to go for a walk whenever and wherever she pleased.

I kept hoping to catch a glimpse of a familiar face from the home, but no one came. Mrs. Smith had started down the next block, so I decided that the best thing to do was to stay with her. I asked the police to call the home, and then to have one of their cars follow us, so that the staff would know where we were. The police did neither. The head nurse never mentioned a call from the police afterward, and they stopped following us as soon as we had walked around the next corner. The police were of no help to me at all. How do they handle themselves in more serious matters?

We arrived back at the home after two hours of walking approximately forty-two blocks in what I was later informed were the worst streets and the toughest neighborhood in the district. At the corner of one street, a group of men checked us out; and then finally the leader said, "No, sir." As I sighed in relief, he remarked,

"All she has on is a watch." The next day, one of the other aides told me that she would never walk around that area, especially with an old lady by the arm, because "They might think she was some rich old lady with her private nurse, and then they'd do a job on you." The head nurse added that she would never walk around there without her husband, and even then she did not like the idea.

Why wasn't someone out looking for us if this was known to be such a dangerous place in which to walk, even during the day? Why did the head nurse lie to me by telling me that Mrs. Smith's sister was coming to pick her up within a few minutes at the entrance of the home? I found out later that the sister never had any intention of coming over at all that afternoon.

Why didn't the head nurse explain to me how to take care of this woman before I became responsible for her? It was easier at the time to send me off on a false pretext, with no explanation, rather than to help me understand Mrs. Smith's mental condition, and perhaps enable me to handle the situation better.

Why was the head nurse so rude and intolerant when my friends, who were supposed to pick me up at 3:00 that afternoon, called the home three times, because they were so worried about my safety? During the first call, the nurse said that Mrs. Smith and I were out walking, and had not yet returned. During the second call, the nurse said, "They still have not returned, and I do not know where they are, but the manager is out looking for them." The third time she said, "Do not call back again, because if they are not back in a few hours, they have probably been abducted!" and hung up.

What story did the head nurse tell the receptionist? The next day she told me I should be ashamed of myself for having taken that old woman through such a dreadful area, and so far. Of course, I had not led Mrs. Smith. I had had no more idea than she did of where we were going, how long we would be gone, what sort of neighborhood we were walking in, or how long our legs would hold out.

Why hadn't someone come to help us when we called

so many times to explain where we were and ask to be picked up? The manager and the head nurse did, in fact, come out in cars looking for us, but only within a three-block radius, when by then, as they knew, we were at least ten blocks away.

Why didn't the taxicab wait and help me settle Mrs. Smith in the car?

Why didn't the police help the way I had asked them to?

Why had I been so helpless? How could a head nurse have put a mentally deranged patient in the hands of an inexperienced aide who was unfamiliar with the patient, and unfamiliar with the surroundings?

THE PROBLEMS

"A nursing home is a place to go and die, and rot away in the process." So wrote one of our many correspondents during our study of nursing homes and health care for the aged. Some people may consider such a statement extravagant, born of a reaction to the condition of old age and its peculiar repulsion for most Americans rather than based on an objective assessment of conditions in the nursing home. Others may write it off as the hysteria of a daughter who cannot bear to see her parent subject to the pain and infirmities that naturally come with old age.

But the comment is typical. Many others reported similar conclusions about the institutions to which one million elderly Americans are consigned. Their criticisms ranged from callous and incompetent staff to shocking drug abuse, from lack of rehabilitative programs to neglect of patients by physicians. We were able to observe many examples of inadequate care in nursing homes where we worked or visited. We were able to compare out observations with those of others who have reported similar problems and abuses in newspapers around the country. That these examples are not isolated incidents, to be found only in a few substandard nursing homes, is suggested by the startling fact that 80 per cent of the nursing homes that receive public tax dollars do not meet even minimal Federal standards.[1]

Clearly some people do receive the care and compassion in nursing homes that they have the right to expect. In addition to letters of outrage, we received equally fervent expressions of gratitude from people whose relatives have found competent health care and a meaningful environment. One family wrote: "We are writing this letter as an official record to state our high opinion of the professional and efficient way you operate the * * * nursing home. To each and every member of the staff, all employees, we want to extend our many thanks for the excellent care and attention given to our husband and father. For all the kind acts, constant supervision and understanding of Mr. A's long illness we again say thanks from the bottom of our hearts."

Everything indicates that such an experience is the exception rather than the norm. Why can't all elderly Americans expect the kind of care that this man received? Is it because they are poor? Because there are too few such institutions? Because their government has not seen fit to insure that their needs are met? Is it because the medical profession has not provided the leadership or support to insure adequate health care for the aged? Or because nursing homes are controlled by a profit-oriented industry that includes profits and losses in its standards of health care and human need? Is it because the elderly themselves do not have the resources to mount a sustained and systematic lobby for better care, while the outrage of their families usually dies with the older relative? Our study attempted to analyze some of the reasons that many older Americans live out their so-called "golden" years in pain and loneliness.

The government has moved toward helping older people pay for the care they need, through Medicare benefits for all persons aged sixty-five and older, and welfare assistance payments (Medicaid) for the medically indigent. But there is evidence that many older people are still unable to afford the price of care. Of the twenty million persons sixty-five and over in the United States, 4.8 million are below the government poverty level and some two million more are too poor to afford necessary medical expenses. Of these nearly seven million people, only 2,050,000 were receiving Old Age Assistance as of April, 1970. Medicaid is designed to help the needy or medically needy, but officials of the Department of Health, Education and Welfare estimate that a low percentage, perhaps less than half, of those eligible for the program are registered. Coinsurance and deductibles under Medicare are severe hardships for many elderly, while gaps in the program—out-of-hospital drugs, for example, are not covered—still leave them with huge bills to pay on their own. Older persons have less than half the income of younger people, while their medical expenses are nearly three times as great. Medical costs fall unevenly, with those least able to pay often incurring larger costs because of inadequate health care in the past.[2]

It is obvious that no single kind of medical treatment facility can meet the needs of the aged. Some need intensive hospital care; others need round-the-clock custodial care; still others need only a pair of younger legs to run out and buy the groceries. Yet there is almost no flexibility in the present system. Hospitals are overcrowded, and so expensive as to place them out of reach for many of the aged. One million elderly people are in some twenty-four thousand nursing homes across the country; but this is only 5 per cent of the aged population, and nursing homes are so crowded and generally provide such miserable care that it is impossible to conceive of their taking care of more people. For the other 95 per cent, the alternatives are few indeed. Home nursing services are costly and hard to find, especially in nonurban areas; community housing is practically nonexistent; anyone who has tried to arrange care for an aged relative knows that all forms of noninstitutional care are woefully lacking. So bad is the situation that an official of the Department of Health, Education and Welfare told us that on any given day 50 per cent of the aged are in the wrong place: if they are in a hospital, they should be in a nursing home; if in a nursing home, they should be at home, and so forth.

For those in nursing homes, little is being done to insure that the elderly receive adequate care even when they can pay for it. The Federal government has so far failed to enforce standards for nursing homes despite overwhelming evidence that many of them are not providing proper care. Results of ineffective standard setting are not always obvious to the casual visitor who may be impressed by the thick carpets in the parlor and the color television set. Rarely does the public take a searching look at the bedrooms, bathrooms, kitchens, and therapy rooms (if any) which are the boundaries of existence for most nursing home patients.

Rarely are the consequences of a lax enforcement policy forced on the national consciousness as they were on January 9, 1970, when a fire in an Ohio nursing home took the lives of thirty-two patients. The tragedy revealed that Medicare standards almost wholly omitted safety provisions. More recently, twenty-five elderly patients in a Maryland nursing home died of salmonella poisoning. Investigation disclosed not only a lack of enforced sanitary food standards, but the failure of physicians and staff to report the epidemic to state health authorities. The tragedy revealed that while doctors attend individual patients in a nursing home, they have neglected the home itself; medical supervision of nursing homes virtually does not exist.

As Congressman David Pryor of Arkansas pointed out after sixteen months of studying nursing homes, "We have turned over the sickest, the most helpless and the most vulnerable patient group in the medical care system to the most loosely controlled and least responsible faction of that system." [3]

The failure to place and accept responsibility is endemic to the entire system of health care for the elderly. Indeed, a major result of this study has been the conclusion that no one group—the government, the nursing home industry, the medical profession—looks on itself as responsible for achieving adequate institutional care for the elderly. Responsibility for nursing homes is spread through at least six Federal agencies among the twenty-two that deal with health services, through at least three agencies in each state, and additional local agencies that have a part in licensing, inspecting, and setting standards. Congressional efforts to upgrade standards by requiring the licensing of nursing home administrators have been diluted, and the nursing home industry now controls the licensing apparatus in most states. There is no one in the Federal bureaucracy responsible for overseeing rehabilitative, or restorative, programs in nursing homes. Training programs for nursing home aides are practically nonexistent and there are few visible efforts to institute them. The list of problems goes on and on.

The bedsores and boredom visible on the bodies and faces of nursing home residents are only symptoms of a national disease. The course of the disease can be traced through government programs that are ill-managed, underfinanced, and fragmented. It can be traced through failure of our national leaders to make a firm commitment to adequate health care for elderly Americans. The U.S. House of Representatives does not yet have a committee specifically assigned to deal with the problems of aging, although the Senate has long had one, and although such a committee seems necessary to protect the interests of the aged, who do not lobby and do not vote as a bloc, and who, as a result usually find that programs that benefit them are the first to go when the Federal budget is squeezed. The disease can be traced through a medical profession that places professional jealousy before professional responsibility, and through a profit-oriented nursing home industry so concerned with cutting costs that it sometimes cuts off lives. It can be traced through a society whose aversion to the very condition of old age, even in the best of circumstances, has resulted in a tragic blindness to the needs of old age, the crushing costs of medical care, and the shattering psychological costs of retirement.

In the pages that follow, we trace this disease through

(1) the history of efforts to enact legislation providing health insurance for Americans; its result in the Medicare and Medicaid programs; and their impact on the nursing home.

(2) the conditions inside the nursing home as shown in Federal standards and licensing; the administrator, the owner, the personnel; the facility; the drugs; and the incentive to live.

(3) alternatives for the elderly outside the nursing home.

2 The Government and Nursing Homes

LEGISLATIVE HISTORY OF NATIONAL HEALTH INSURANCE

What is he like, this old man who stares vacantly at the television set in a nursing home, or who steps slowly and painfully into the bus, or who, if he is fortunate, sits down to Sunday dinner with a swarm of grandchildren? He is, first of all, likely to be a woman; after the age of sixty-five the longer life expectancy of women begins to tell, and less than 45 per cent of the aged are men. Of the women, slightly more than half are widowed; of the aged women who earn any income at all, half bring home less than one thousand dollars a year.

The aged person is a settled person. He is much less likely to move than a younger person, and is much more likely to own his home. Unfortunately, his home may be the only wealth he has; the median income for an aged man is less than half that for the total population. With a low and probably fixed income and assets such as his home that cannot easily be converted into cash, he is especially vulnerable to a number of dangers. The property tax is one; catastrophic or chronic medical expenses are another.

In 1962, only 3 per cent of aged couples incurred no medical costs whatsoever. On the average, the person over sixty-five spends more than twice as much for medical care as the person under sixty-five, although he has only half the income. Almost seven out of ten aged couples who reported hospital costs in 1962 were faced with bills over five hundred dollars; the figure has risen substantially since then. Compared with the younger population, the noninstitutionalized aged person is twice as likely to have a chronic illness and almost three times as likely to have days on which he must restrict his activity because of illness. Forty-four out of one thousand aged people receive some form of home medical care, and half of these need it constantly. A man or woman over sixty-five is 36 per cent more likely to go to a doctor than a younger person.[1]

These were the conditions when Medicare and Medicaid set out on the final leg of their legislative journey. Federal health insurance for the aged was a long time coming, and when it came was long overdue. In the second decade of the century, Theodore Roosevelt planned to make national health insurance a major plank of the Progressive Party platform, but the First World War broke out and deflected attention from domestic needs. The pattern continued; time and again interest in national health insurance arose, only to be met with major crisis after major crisis—the Depression, the Second World War, the turbulent first years of the Cold War—and replaced at the bottom of a stack of priorities. With the important exceptions of the Social Security Act (1935) and the Hill-Burton Hospital Survey and Construction Act (1946), Federal policy toward the aged and toward medical care changed little until 1950.

Foreign and domestic crises alone cannot explain the country's delay in enacting legislation to help the aged meet their enormous medical costs. From the beginning, the medical professions, led by the American Medical Association, pitted their formidable political power against attempts to establish a national health insurance. Their arguments were familiar—cries of socialized medicine, of interference with the privacy of the doctor-patient relationship, of a crippling of the quality of medical care—but they were strong. Especially because of the Depression, when a people starved for leadership turned with their trust to physicians, who had always been leading community figures, the AMA was enormously influential. The AMA and its allies—the American Hospital Association, the American Nursing Home Association, and others—never lost a legislative battle until 1950. In that year the Democratic Congress established an Old Age Assistance program, under which aged persons on welfare could apply state and Federal funds directly to their medical costs. It was a step in the right direction, but it did little about the old person not on welfare who, although he could meet routine living expenses, was unable to cope with the sudden, high costs of illness.

The turning point came in 1955, when the American Federation of Labor and the Congress of Industrial Organizations merged. Separately, each had been a powerful supporter of national health insurance, and together they formed a lobby whose power could rival that of the AMA. In 1956, the new labor organization tested its muscle, and, over the opposition of the AMA, won passage of a new Social Security benefit for permanently disabled people over the age of fifty. (Eventually, Congress was to remove the age limit, due to the program's low cost and big success.) And although the benefit was minor, the fact that its passage was the AMA's second defeat made it a major event of the year. After a monotony of defeats, advocates of a national health insurance program were optimistic once more.

One other event occurred that most people did not notice at the time. William Reidy, a staff member of the Senate Committee on Labor and Public Welfare, was convinced that the problems of the elderly were economically and socially affecting the rest of the population as well, and he suggested a Senate subcommittee on aging. He chose Senator John Kennedy as a likely crusader. Although Kennedy liked the idea, he was too involved with his subcommittee on labor to start a new subcommittee. However, Kennedy did get together with Senator Lister Hill of Alabama, and the two cosponsored an encompassing bill that dealt with many of the problems of the aged. This Senior Citizens Opportunity and Security bill had been drafted by Wilbur Cohen, who had left HEW to become a professor of public welfare administration at the University of Michigan. In June, 1956, the two senators introduced the bill which aroused no interest and never even came to a vote. However, one result of their action was a thirty-thousand dollar grant for the study of the problems of the aged and the aging; the subcommittee that took over the grant, under the direction of Wilbur Cohen, compiled a ten-volume report, which was subsequently filed away at the Library of Congress. This subcommittee was to expand into the Senate Special Committee on Aging.

Late in 1956, Nelson Cruikshank (then the Social Security director of the AFL-CIO) collaborated with Wilbur Cohen, I. S. Falk, and Robert Ball (a top man in the Social Security Administration) on a bill that was similar to the "beneficiaries" bill.

> Like its predecessor, the bill gave the elderly sixty days of hospitalization, but it went on to cover the costs of surgery and of care in nursing homes. Hospitals, doctors, and nursing homes were free to join the plan or stay out of it, and patients were free to choose any of the physicians or institutions participating. In addition, it was made clear that "nothing in the provisions of the bill . . . shall be construed to give the Secretary of Health, Education and Welfare [who was to administer the program] supervision or control over, first, the practice of medicine or the manner in which medical services are provided; second, the details of administration or operation of hospitals or nursing homes; or, third, the selection, tenure, or compensation of hospital or nursing-home personnel." The benefits were to be paid for by increasing the amount of income on which Social Security taxes were levied from $4,200 to $6,000 (enough to allow a sweetener in the form of a ten per cent increase in payments to everyone covered by Social Security) and by increasing the tax rate itself by one-half of one per cent for both employees and employers. These changes, an H.E.W. actuary reported, would produce enough revenue to pay for the annual cost of the program—around eight hundred million dollars.[2]

The four men went to the House Committee on Ways and Means, which handles tax legislation, and tried to interest the top representatives in their bill. The fourth man in seniority, Aime Forand of Rhode Island, was finally persuaded to endorse the bill. Late in 1957, Forand submitted the bill to Congress, but too late to get any action on it. The introduction of this bill began the last of a long series of legislative struggles for a national health insurance. In the eight years that followed, the bill was revised a total of eighty times.

The AMA's reaction in 1958 was to set up a Joint Council to Improve the Health Care of the Aged, made up of the AMA, the American Hospital Association, the American Dental Association, and the American Nursing Home Association.

> The title turned out to be a misnomer, for the council's chief conclusion was that the health care of the aged didn't need improving. Not only were the aged getting top-notch medical care, it reported, but they were far better off economically and in most other respects than younger people were. Indeed, the council urged everyone to consider not the problems of the elderly, but their opportunities.[3]

Using this strategy, the AMA testified against the Forand bill at the hearings in June, 1958.

Nelson Cruikshank testified in favor of the bill, pointing out that the alternative health insurance programs that had been in effect for some time were not meeting the needs of the elderly. Voluntary insurance plans required their participants to pay much higher premiums after they retired if the insurance was to continue. Commercial insurance companies designed their plans to exclude old retirees, in order to concentrate on the younger workers, the "better risks." This left the sick and the elderly in the hands of the nonprofit programs, such as Blue Cross and Blue Shield.

Cruikshank argued that it was imperative that the Federal health insurance provisions for the elderly described in the Forand bill be instituted immediately. He was backed up by the American Nurses Association, the Group Health Association of America, the American Public Welfare Association, the National Farmers' Union, and the National Association of Social Workers.

The Forand bill hearings magnified the increasing polarization between the opposing sides of the national health insurance issue. A very real and obvious fight between organized medicine and the labor unions had developed. At the end of the hearings, the Ways and Means Committee concluded that no further action could be taken on the bill until more background on the problem had been gathered. HEW was given the task of gathering this information.

Senator John Kennedy's increasing interest in the plight of the elderly was shown in a speech called "A Bill of Rights for Our Elder Citizens" that he gave to the Senate on August 19, 1958. That speech, along with concerted efforts of Senators Hill and McNamara of Michigan, resulted in the setting up of the Sub-committee on Problems of the Aged and Aging in February, 1959.

Although Congress did nothing further with the Forand bill in 1958, it approved a Social Security bene-fit increase (and a subsequent increase in the taxable wage base) independent of the bill that fall. Forand's bill had called for these changes; when they were imple-mented without his bill, he was able to focus all his effort on the issue of health insurance for the aged when he introduced his bill again in 1959.

The overall situation looked good for passage of the bill in 1959. Congressional support was improving, due to Democratic gains during the 1958 midterm elections. The new Senate Subcommittee on Problems of the Aged and Aging was beginning to attract more public interest with hearings held around the country. During these public hearings, many old people lined up to speak; their main complaint was poor medical care. Consistent with this complaint were the findings of the HEW study of the background of the problem:

> The rising cost of medical care, and particularly of hos-pital care, over the past decade has been felt by persons of all ages. Older persons have greater than average med-ical care needs. As a group they use about two-and-a-half times as much general hospital care as the average for persons under age 65, and they have special need for long-term institutional care. Their incomes are generally con-siderably lower than those of the rest of the population, and in many cases are either fixed or declining in amount. They have less opportunity than employed persons to spread the cost burden through health insurance. A larger proportion of the aged than of other persons must turn to public assistance for payment of their medical bills or

rely on "free" care from hospitals and physicians. Because both the number and proportion of older persons in the population are increasing, a satisfactory solution to the problem of paying for adequate medical care for the aged will become more rather than less important.[4]

As advocates of the Forand bill became more optimistic, the AMA became more alarmed. Congressional hearings were held on the bill in 1959, but again no legislative action was taken. As the problems of the aged became more and more widely publicized, however, there was a feeling that something was bound to happen soon.

Public pressure and clamor for legislative action on the health insurance issue created an exciting political climate in 1960, an election year. The Forand bill was defeated twice that year in its original form, and once in a version that provided hospital benefits only. At the same time, however, the Ways and Means Committee rejected the Republican alternative, which provided Federal grants to states to help subsidize private health insurance programs for the low-income elderly. By now the issue was not whether the elderly needed Federal help but rather how the money should be channeled to them. The Ways and Means Committee rejected Social Security financing and private company financing; the health care issue was at a deadlock.

Then Wilbur Mills, chairman of the Ways and Means Committee, introduced a compromise bill for expansion of the "medical vendors" payment program of 1950, using Federal matching funds to pay for state medical care for the aged. Social Security was left out of the picture. The bill was quickly approved by the Committee and passed by the House three weeks later. Proponents of the Forand bill were hopeful that a health insurance amendment would be attached to the bill in the Senate.

Senator Robert Kerr of Oklahoma, a wealthy and powerful man on the Senate Finance Committee, who was also up for re-election, recognized the potential of the Mills bill. He consulted with Wilbur Cohen, and together they drew up a new bill that incorporated much of the Mills bill but also covered those he termed "medically indigent"—the elderly who can pay for everything but their medical expenses. This Kerr-Mills bill was the forerunner of Medicaid.

Attacking the new Kerr-Mills proposal as inadequate to deal with the problems of the aged, Senators John Kennedy and Clinton P. Anderson drafted a new health insurance bill that went even further than the Forand bill. It provided 120 days of hospital care, 240 days of nursing home care, and 360 home health visits by visiting nurses each year.

Although Cohen realized that the Democrats still favored financing health insurance through Social Security, he knew that if they were presented with the choice of either the Kennedy-Anderson bill or the Kerr-Mills bill, they would settle for the latter. He proved to be right; the Senate defeated the Kennedy-Anderson bill 51–44, and the Kerr-Mills proposal swept through by a vote of 91–2. The Senate-House conference committee approved the bill two days later with few changes, and in mid-September, 1960, the Kerr-Mills bill became law.

A long-planned White House Conference on the Aging was held early in 1961. It had been organized during Eisenhower's administration and three officials who had ranked high in that administration publicly endorsed the Kerr-Mills program. The general trend of the gathering was toward health insurance through Social Security, since the Secretary of HEW, Arthur Flemming, had relied on the advice of Nelson Cruikshank in arranging the Conference.

Following the White House Conference, President Kennedy sent a special health message to Congress. Soon after, he also sent Congress a new health bill.

The new Medicare bill provided for ninety days of hospital care . . . outpatient diagnostic services . . . a hundred and eighty days of nursing or other health specialists. Its provisions were available to all Social Security beneficiaries sixty-five or older, about fourteen million people. The annual cost of the bill was estimated at a billion and a half dollars—including federal grants for the construction of medical school facilities and for loans to medical students, both of which the A.M.A. opposed. The cost was to be paid by an increase of one-quarter of one per cent in the Social Security tax on both employees and employers.[5]

Senator Anderson sponsored the bill in the Senate, and Representative Cecil King of California managed the bill in the House. Hearings were held on the bills, but again, the only result was a further division between the opposing sides.

Then a series of events occurred which delayed the Medicare bill until 1962. First, the Democrats had lost some seats in Congress with Kennedy's narrow victory; there was not enough support on the Committee or in the House to risk bringing the bill to a vote. Second, America was going through a mild recession, and priority was given to antirecession bills. Most important, Kennedy was faced with several touchy foreign affairs problems during the next few months, such as the Bay of Pigs incident, the Berlin Wall crisis, a meeting with Khrushchev, and increasing Communist pressure in Laos. Kennedy therefore decided to wait until 1962 for the big Medicare push.

Meanwhile, the AMA took this opportunity to make it clear to the public where the organization stood on the health insurance issue. Through pamphlets, speeches, radio and television broadcasts and announcements, the AMA flooded the public with anti-Medicare propaganda. The AMA also organized its own full-time political action group, the American Medical Political Action Committee (AMPAC), which concentrated its efforts on encouraging the states to implement the new Kerr-Mills program.

Another voice against the Administration's Medicare proposal was from the insurance companies, who challenged the estimated costs of Medicare. Both the commercial carriers and the nonprofit Blue Shield-Blue Cross programs began to develop their own low-cost programs for the elderly, in an attempt to come up with a non-Federal answer to the problem.

On behalf of Medicare, a National Council of Senior Citizens (NCSC) was established, consisting mostly of pensioners from labor unions, as well as people from nonprofit retirement centers, church groups, and the like. One by one, community organizations came over to the side of the NCSC. The American Nurses Association, the American Hospital Association, and the American Public Health Association all broke with the AMA to endorse the King-Anderson bill—or at least to admit that Federal health insurance was greatly needed, no matter where the money came from.

1962 seemed like the year for Medicare. Kennedy was prepared to push Medicare through; votes in favor of the bill were supposedly gathering in the Ways and Means Committee. Republicans in the House and the Senate began to shift to the camp that favored financing through Social Security, with the option for private insurance. Even the AMA admitted that Federal subsidies channeled through Blue Cross and Blue Shield might be necessary. The NCSC held a huge rally in Madison Square Garden on May 20, 1962. President Kennedy made a personal appearance and spoke to a crowd of nearly twenty thousand old people, while the event was broadcast live across the nation. The AMA's response was to televise, two days later, a speech in Madison Square Garden by Dr. Annis, the head of their speaker's bureau. Dr. Annis spoke to an empty stadium—to emphasize the AMA's lonely fight against Medicare.

A week later, the Ways and Means Committee began executive sessions on Medicare, but after three weeks the issue was again stymied. Senator Anderson wanted to break the deadlock by attaching the bill as a rider to a House-passed tax measure pending in the Senate. But he was forced to compromise with Senator Jacob Javits of New York, who wanted to put his own version of the tax measure to a vote, which would bring a vote on the original measure before it could be amended with Anderson's Medicare proposal. The compromise resulted in an Anderson-Javits Amendment to the House-passed welfare bill presented to the floor on June 29, 1962. But 1962 was an election year, and the Senate was operating cautiously; after two weeks of tense lobbying and deliberation, the whole bill was defeated. President Kennedy was furious and vowed to make Medicare a key issue for the fall elections. The attempt to slip Medicare

through by attaching it to a much needed welfare bill
had only resulted in the defeat of the whole measure.

In early 1963, public pressure for Medicare was growing again.

> . . . A Senate report on the Kerr-Mills program showed
> that it was working not in thirty-eight states—already a
> mysterious decline from the A.M.A.'s claim of forty-six
> the year before—but in twenty-four. Of these, New York,
> Massachusetts, Michigan, and California were getting
> ninety per cent of all federal funds being distributed—
> chiefly because they were the only states able and willing
> to match government grants in any significant amounts.
> Where the Kerr-Mills program was operating, the report
> continued, it was usually operating in a very limited way.
> In March, a total of eighty-eight thousand people, or
> about one-half of one per cent of the country's aged pop-
> ulation, had received some form of assistance, and more
> often than not the assistance hadn't amounted to much.[6]

Reports showed that the size of the elderly population
was still rapidly growing, from twelve million, or eight
per cent of the total population, in 1950; to seventeen
and a half million, or 9.4 per cent of the population, in
1963. And the cost of hospital care was still rising, from
twenty-nine dollars a day in 1960, to forty dollars a day
in 1963. The Blue Cross-Blue Shield plans for low-cost
health insurance for the elderly turned out to be empty
promises. The NCSC was growing steadily, and the
Senate Special Committee on Aging was gaining more
interest and pressure for Medicare with public hearings
around the nation. The Administration presented a new
version of the bill, revised to cover an additional three
million people over sixty-five who were not Social Security beneficiaries and who were not covered under
previous bills. Although President Kennedy was eager to
seize the opportunity to get Medicare through, the Ways
and Means Committee was forced to devote most of
1963 to other pressing issues, such as civil rights, the
nuclear test ban treaty, and an omnibus tax reform
measure. It was not until mid-November that the Committee was able to hold further hearings on Medicare.
The time was right, the public was anxious, the session
was getting heated, and things were looking good for
Medicare when ". . . the committee's chief counsel hur-

ried into the room and whispered something to Chairman Mills. Turning pale, Mills interrupted the proceedings to announce that President Kennedy had been shot, and then adjourned the hearings." [7]

The swell of public support for everything that Kennedy had stood for or believed in that arose after his death was emotional and massive. President Lyndon Johnson gathered this support behind Medicare, for he was as eager as Kennedy had been to get the bill through.

But in 1964, Chairman Mills of the Ways and Means Committee was still holding out against Medicare during executive sessions, using the bill's estimated costs as his excuse. Before the bill could be defeated in committee, Representative King pleaded for a delay. Two weeks later, a Social Security benefits increase (H.R. 11865) was approved by the Committee, passed by the House, and sent on to the Senate Finance Committee.

There, supporters of the Medicare proposal, in an attempt to avoid committee defeat or deadlock in the House, attached Medicare to the newly passed tax bill. This time the strategy worked. On September 2, 1964, the King-Anderson bill was passed as an amendment to H.R. 11865, and for the first time in American history, the Senate passed a government health insurance plan.

The next step was to persuade the House to accept the amended bill in the House-Senate conference committee. A tacit agreement had been made that the Social Security tax increase would not exceed 10 per cent. However, with the 5 per cent increase on the cash benefits in the Social Security bill, the 10 per cent ceiling was not high enough to add sufficient funds for Medicare. The Republicans on the conference committee insisted that the tax increase for the cash benefits was necessary, while the Democrats fought to include Medicare. Mills called an unexpected vote on the cash increase amendments without Medicare, but surprisingly the proposal was defeated. The issue was again at a deadlock; Mills adjourned the session with nothing accomplished.

Johnson's open determination to get Medicare passed helped to give him a landslide victory in the 1964 election.

An analysis of the election returns showed that twenty-two per cent of the vote had been cast by people over the age of sixty, two million of whom had switched from the Republican column to the Democratic. And though seven of the ten states with the highest percentage of elderly voters were traditionally Republican, all ten went to the Democrats.[8]

1965 had to be the year. Political support was good, the political climate was getting better, the public trusted the Social Security system, the economy was blooming, and the President was determined. The King-Anderson bill was given top priority and was the first bill submitted that year in both the Senate and the House. Hearings were held before the Ways and Means Committee, at which the AMA proposed an alternative, "Eldercare." The AMA claimed that Eldercare "would provide federal and state grants, under the provisions of the Kerr-Mills program, to subsidize private health-insurance policies for old people who wanted them," [9] and actually offered more benefits than Medicare. The subsequent publicity that Eldercare received backfired on the AMA, for Chairman Mills realized that Medicare would have to be expanded if the nation's elderly were to be pleased. But there were still the AMA and the insurance companies to appease. Using three different proposals for health care, Mills meshed them into a political work of art that would satisfy everyone.

Mills proposed first to expand the Kerr-Mills program to take care of the indigent elderly (Medicaid), second to have Medicare take care of the middle-income elderly, paying for hospital, nursing home, and home health care. Finally, to please the AMA and the insurance companies, Mills proposed to use a bill drafted by Representative Byrnes of Wisconsin that created a Federal voluntary insurance program that would pay for doctors' fees in and out of hospitals. Everything was complete.

The Mills bill swept through the Ways and Means Committee on March 23, 1965. Later that afternoon, President Johnson gave approval to the five-hundred-million-dollar increase in the budget that would be necessary if the bill passed. On April 8, the bill swept through the House by a vote of 313–115.

This left the Senate as the final obstacle. On nation-wide TV President Johnson elicited from Chairman Byrd of the Senate Finance Committee a promise to set up "prompt" and "thorough" hearings on the bill. The hearings were held in late April, and the Committee went into executive session to prepare a version of the House bill. On June 17, Senator Long of Louisiana sauntered into the conference room, and, with only thirteen of the twenty-five Committee members present, quickly proposed and called a vote on two amendments to the bill.

> The first of them, he said, would make Medicare's provisions unlimited, in order to take care of what he called "catastrophic illness." (Since a ten-minute illness can be catastrophic for the person suffering it, it was assumed that Long was using the term to describe long-term illnesses that were catastrophically expensive.) The second was designed to pay for this open-end feature by adding, on top of the increase in Social Security taxes, a sliding scale of deductibles, or amounts to be paid by the patients themselves, based on their incomes.[10]

The amendments, so unreasonable that they were probably meant to kill the bill, were passed with two proxy votes, 8–7. But the winning proxy vote was later invalidated; in a new vote the next day, both amendments were defeated. Senator Hartke proposed a thirty-day, ten-dollar-a-day deductible amendment, which was passed, and the following day, Long added a similar amendment for thirty more days.

The bill was finally approved by the Senate Finance Committee and sent to the Senate with seventy-five committee amendments. Long, appointed floor manager of the bill, almost managed to kill it again. Three days, 513 amendments, and an additional one and a half billion dollars later, the bill passed the Senate, 68–21. In the Senate-House conference committee that followed, Mills managed to bring the bill down in size, and the final bill was approved by the House on July 27 and by the Senate on July 28, 1965.

Thus, after fifty years of almost constant debate and

struggle, America had earned health insurance protection for her aged.

MEDICARE, MEDICAID, AND THE NURSING HOME

The American Medical Association lost its battle against national health insurance, but its powerful opposition had an effect nonetheless. The Mills compromise that brought forth Medicare was not the orderly outcome of a well-developed national health policy but was designed to mollify contending forces. Limited in its own provisions, it is also separated from other health services programs, for which there is no single agency in the Federal government responsible. Compromise has meant piecemeal programs and a diffusion of responsibility, with a consequent weakening of efforts to enforce standards of quality.

Nowhere is this fragmentation more evident than in the case of nursing homes, for which more than six agencies in the Department of Health, Education and Welfare alone have a morsel of responsibility. The division between health insurance under Medicare and medical assistance payments under Medicaid, both of which include nursing home benefits, meant the establishment of different standards and different administrative bureaucracies comprising numerous and overlapping agencies that deal with nursing homes. Thus, a single nursing home may now be inspected under three sets of standards—state licensing codes, Medicare standards, and Medicaid standards. The inspectors are usually local health department employees who are supervised by state surveyors who report to a Federal agency. Responsibility is passed up and down the chain of command without forceful guidance or final enforcement power fixed at any one point. In the absence of one agency clearly designated as responsible, and capable of assuming that responsibility, the public interest in insuring high-quality care in nursing homes has been frustrated.

MEDICARE AND THE NURSING HOME

The passage of Medicare and Medicaid in 1965 marked the beginning of the first real involvement of the Federal government in nursing homes, although the Hill-Burton Hospital Survey and Construction Act of 1946 provided funds to assist in the building of nursing homes. The Medicare bill provided three basic forms of assistance: automatic hospital insurance for citizens sixty-five and over; payment for treatment in an "Extended Care Facility" after leaving the hospital; and payment for home nursing care. Ironically, two of the three forms of assistance were unavailable, for all practical purposes: six out of seven Medicare recipients live in areas where home nursing care simply does not exist, and the Extended Care Facility (ECF) was a totally new concept in health care developed by a harried Congress that for a moment lost sight of reality.

The story of the ECF shows the effects of the many political compromises necessary to get the Medicare bill passed. In lobbying against Medicare, the AMA and other professional groups argued that passage of the bills would flood the nation's hospitals with more elderly patients than could possibly be handled. Moreover, the AMA claimed, hospital rates were so high that any significant influx of patients would make the costs of Medicare soar out of sight. It was in response to these arguments that the House Ways and Means Committee, with the help of the AMA, developed the concept of the ECF. The ECF was to provide short-term post-hospital care for patients who no longer needed intensive hospital treatment but who did need continued institutional care during recuperation.[1] Few such facilities actually existed; only some six hundred hospitals had special wards or wings for convalescent care.[2] Those who conceived the ECF envisioned an expansion of this kind of in-hospital facility, but their dream bubble promptly burst.

At the outset, there was confusion as to the exact purpose and definition of the ECF benefits. To the public, the term "extended" meant a long period of time although, in fact, ECF meant a short-term extension of hospital care. In the eyes of the community, a nursing home was a place where the elderly went when they had nowhere else to go, and where they received custodial care until they died. Certification as an ECF did little to change the image of the nursing home. Therefore, the public was led to believe that Medicare provided for long-term nursing home care when actually it provided for only one-hundred days of very limited benefits. The patient had to have spent at least three days in a hospital prior to admission; he had to be admitted to the ECF within fourteen days of discharge from the hospital; he had to need and receive skilled nursing treatment for the same illness for which he was hospitalized; and he had to have rehabilitative potential.[3]

Even the Social Security Administration was confused about the role of the extended care facility. The chief actuary, Robert Myers, who drew up the cost estimates for the program, assumed that the ECF benefit would replace the last few days normally spent in a hospital. For example, if the average hospital stay for a person sixty-five or over was fifteen days, Myers assumed that the last three days would now be spent in an ECF. Others within the Social Security Administration, particularly those responsible for explaining Medicare benefits to the public, assumed that the ECF benefit was in addition to the normal hospital stay.[4]

The semantic confusion surrounding the ECF was cut through ingeniously. Realizing that most people assumed that an ECF was a nursing home, and realizing that the Medicare program needed many such facilities quickly, the Social Security Administration decided to let nursing homes double as Extended Care Facilities, providing convalescent care, which would be covered by Medicare, and custodial care, which would not be covered.[5] So the Social Security Administration (SSA) established standards for Extended Care Facilities and began to search for suitable nursing homes. The standards were none too stringent; the AMA had successfully argued that if high standards were set so few institutions would qualify, the program would be useless. So it was with confidence that the Social Security Administration sent out thirteen thousand letters to the nation's nursing homes inviting them to participate in the new Medicare ECF program.

SSA officials were shocked to find that the number of qualified homes did not begin to approach the number required. The conditions for participation in the Medicare program were to be described later by the staff of the Senate Finance Committee as "tightly drafted with reasonably high-quality standards." [6] They included provisions for twenty-four-hour nursing service, a nursing care plan based on personalized, daily needs of individual patients, and proper dietary supervision.[7] The startling revelation was that only a fraction of the nursing homes—around 740 out of 13,000—were able to meet these conditions. The Social Security Administration was thrown into a panic and therefore made a foolish decision. It responded to the shortage of qualified Extended Care Facilities not by instituting a massive drive to help or force them to come up to standards but by ignoring the standards altogether.[8]

STANDARDS AND ENFORCEMENT

Hospital benefits for Medicare went into effect on July 1, 1966, with extended care benefits scheduled to go into effect six months later. Projections indicated a need for twenty-five hundred certified Extended Care Facilities by January, 1967. The Social Security Administration, with little time to come up with enough facilities to handle the expected hospital overload, drew up conditions of participation and sent out letters to over thirteen thousand nursing homes inviting them to join the program. The Secretary of HEW reported to Congress in his First Annual Report on Medicare that:

> . . . by December, 1966, nearly 6,000 facilities had filed applications, on-site surveys were being completed, and the other steps in the certification process were well underway. . . . By January 1, 1967, when the extended care benefit provisions went into effect, approximately 2,800 facilities were in substantial compliance with the conditions of participation. By July 31, 1967, as a result of the assistance provided by state agencies, an additional 1,400 facilities had been approved for participation. This

brought the total number of participating extended care facilities to 4,160.[9]

The Secretary's report does not convey exactly what happened. By December, 1966, the Social Security Administration was desperate, according to those who witnessed the scene from the vantage point of the Department of HEW and from Capitol Hill. The SSA sent frantic messages to the regional offices and state agencies asking them to reconsider some of the nursing homes previously rejected as substandard, and to send in as many certifications as they could. The SSA was already certifying some substandard homes as being in "substantial" compliance. Now it waived all standards and created the category of "conditional" compliance, which included even facilities that did not have a qualified charge nurse for each tour of duty. In a letter to state agencies on December 16, 1966, Arthur E. Hess, Director of the SSA Bureau of Health Insurance, wrote, "For cases which have been withdrawn but which could now qualify under the 'Conditional approval' concept, the state agency should attempt to secure new applications and process them as expeditiously as possible." [10]

By July, 1967, only 740 of the certified Extended Care Facilities met the full conditions of participation; 3,210 were considered in "substantial" compliance; another 210 were certified under "conditional approval." [11]

However "tightly drafted" the standards were in other respects, their provisions for physical environment were geared to accommodate older institutions that did not meet newer Hill-Burton standards for construction of hospitals. These standards were offered simply as "guidelines" and were specifically entrusted to the "discretion" of the local inspectors who were instructed to evaluate facilities "in light of community need for service," rather than in light of patient need for safety.[12] Thus doorways, passageways, and stairwells were only to be "wide enough for easy evacuation of patients," not "wide enough to permit a hospital bed to be rolled through them." Specific fire safety regulations were omitted entirely.* As far as existing institutions were concerned,

* For fuller discussion of fire and safety standards see Chapter 3, Section 2.

the physical environment standards consisted of a huge grandfather clause, and no provisions were made for systematic improvement of outdated facilities.

The staffing requirements, in which many homes proved deficient, were hardly more than minimal. For example, the ECF was required to have "at least one registered professional nurse or qualified licensed practical nurse who is a graduate of a State-approved school of practical nursing on duty at all times and in charge of the nursing activities during each tour of duty." [13] While this requirement was meant to apply to the nursing home providing "intensive" nursing care, it would seem reasonable that any nursing home charged with the care of aged patients should provide twenty-four-hour nursing service. However, this service has proved to be one of the major deficiencies of nursing homes applying for participation in the Medicare program.

The number of nursing homes certified as Extended Care Facilities which progressed from "substantial" to "full" compliance ratings is not impressive. In the course of a year, from July, 1968, to July, 1969, only twenty-four additional nursing homes were rated in full compliance (1,350 in 1968; 1,374 in 1969). Nursing homes in substantial compliance still constituted the vast majority of all homes certified, and these increased at a faster rate than those in full compliance (3,340 in 1968; 3,402 in 1969). The Secretary of HEW reported to Congress that "conditional certifications" granted in January, 1967, expired as of April 1, 1968. Of the 250 facilities, he said, over 200 had met the requirements for regular certification, while "others have withdrawn as providers or have had their participation terminated." [14] The Senate Finance Committee staff reported, however, that ten nursing homes continued under conditional approval as of July, 1968.[15] None have been reported since that time.

The staff of the Senate Finance Committee recommended in its report of February, 1970, that the category of substantial compliance be removed and that only those homes fully meeting the standards receive Federal funds.[16] The staff hoped that more stringent enforcement of standards, together with the threat of cutting off funds, would increase the pressure on nursing homes to comply. The reasoning was that it did not pay homes to comply if they could get Federal funds without instituting improvements that might be costly. The staff felt that the nursing homes had had ample time to make improvements, that taxpayers' money was being wasted, and that it was unconscionable for Medicare to continue to give a veneer of respectability to shoddy facilities. In light of the conditions to which the staff was responding, its recommendation seems mild, but the Social Security Administration continues to allow homes in substantial compliance to participate in the program. On June 15, 1970, the SSA reported 4,656 Extended Care Facilities, of which 1,274 were in full compliance and 3,382 were in substantial compliance.[17] The only observable change is semantic: homes in the substantial compliance category are now said to have "correctable deficiencies." There is no more assurance than before that the deficiencies will in fact be corrected.

As of December, 1969, the highest number of deficiencies, 37 per cent, occurred in the social services requirement for Extended Care Facilities which states that there must be a social worker or staff member trained in social work to coordinate community resources to meet the patients' social and emotional needs. The next most frequent deficiency—29 per cent of the homes—was in physical environment, or facility construction problems. Seventeen per cent of the nursing homes did not have even one registered or licensed practical nurse on duty at all times. Fifteen per cent failed to meet dietary requirements, and 13 per cent did not keep adequate clinical records—an important omission, since the maintenance of proper records is essential to the provision of proper care.[18] All these certified nursing homes were receiving Federal funds.

In 1969, more than two hundred nursing homes withdrew from the Medicare program rather than correct their deficiencies; only sixteen withdrew "involuntarily," under compulsion by the SSA. This small number of terminations required by the Federal government does not imply rigid enforcement measures.

It is difficult to determine just when a nursing home in substantial compliance must move into full compliance in order to continue participating in the Medicare program. SSA regulations call for inspections of all homes every year, and inspections of substantial compliance homes every nine months. The SSA, however, does not check whether inspections follow this schedule. Several correspondents reported that there were no inspections during an entire year in homes where they worked. Morris Levy, Assistant Director of the Division of State Operations in SSA, told us that homes could not remain in substantial compliance indefinitely. In the absence of clear rules for terminating certification, it appears that homes do in fact continue with correctable deficiencies.

The Social Security Administration regulations leave termination to the discretion of inspectors, providing only the most general guidelines for a finding of noncompliance. If the nursing home

> has deficiencies of such character as to seriously limit the capacity of the institution to render adequate care or to place health and safety of individuals in jeopardy, and consultation to institution has demonstrated that there is no early prospect of such significant improvement as to establish substantial compliance as of a later beginning date, or after a previous period or part thereof for which the institution was certified under circumstances outlined in 405.1105(b), there is a lack of progress toward a removal of deficiencies which the State agency finds are adverse to the health and safety of individuals being served.[19]

The language used is so vague that it is meaningless. "Seriously," "adequate," "early," "significant," "substantial"—these are words that an inspector can interpret any way he chooses.

Medicare inspectors, and presumably the Social Security Administration itself, have managed to justify their refusals to crack down on nursing homes that violate government health and safety standards. In an interview, Mamie Dailey, a Medicare inspector in Maryland, said that she was reluctant to deny certification because she preferred to remain in contact with the homes in order to help them conform to basic requirements.[20] While Miss Dailey herself may be successful in helping homes meet the standards, there is little to suggest that the Social Security Administration and Medicare inspectors as a whole have encouraged nursing homes to comply with the law. Without the threat of closing off funds, there is little reason for them to do so.

INSPECTIONS

When Medicare was enacted, Congress decided to entrust the task of certifying nursing homes to the states. Some states, meaning usually the state health department, in turn transfer the responsibility to local county or city health or welfare departments. Local fire and sanitation departments may also inspect for safety and sanitary conditions. The problem of communication and coordination in this system has not worked to facilitate the process of upgrading nursing homes; there is no regulation at the Federal level requiring such coordination. The welfare department may continue placing clients in a home even though health inspectors find the home substandard, so that one agency may nullify the efforts of another.[21]

There are between 850 and 900 state health department surveyors who inspect Extended Care Facilities and 5,000 to 6,000 local employees with some responsibilities for inspection. The Social Security Administration has only a small corps of eight or ten employees who attempt to follow up these inspections. Medicaid surveyors are not currently checked by any Federal officials to see if they are performing their duties satisfactorily.[22] Beginning January 1, 1971, an attempt will be made to establish procedures to evaluate the level of a surveyor's performance so that he can be a "nationally certified and recognized health facilities surveyor."

These efforts are being made under the Public Health Service's Facilities Survey Improvement Program. A prerequisite for surveyor certification will be attendance at a training course in surveying. The Public Health Service first offered such courses in March, 1970, and have since trained forty-five people—thirty-three state

Medicare surveyors and twelve Federal officials engaged in administering Medicare programs. By June 30, 1971, more than 300 people are expected to have completed the course—a far cry from the total number of people involved in inspections. The Public Health Service pays the operating costs of the course, while the SSA pays travel and per diem costs for the surveyors. Title XI funds can be used for such training courses. No Medicaid surveyor has yet attended the institutes, though plans are being made to include them.

More serious than the difficulty of coordinating and training nursing home inspectors is the failure of the Federal government to provide strong leadership and backing for local and state surveyors. Since the beginning of the program, when the SSA urged state inspectors to "reconsider" substandard homes for Medicare, the pattern was set for an inspection process that systematically ignores violations. An HEW employee in Illinois, Raymond Whitener, wrote Congressman David Pryor: "At the beginning of the Medicare program, practically all nursing homes were blanketed in as approved nursing homes and from that day to this we have never had the courage to take away the approval of these substandard facilities." [23] Needless to say, they should have had the courage.

The reaction of Miss Dailey is indicative of the attitude of many state inspectors. She noted that the ultimate step of closing nursing homes is avoided because usually neither the homes nor the state has an alternative to offer the patients. This points again to the helplessness of the elderly patient who may be forced to choose between an inferior home or no home at all.

Local inspectors may be subject to pressure either from officials who fear a shortage of nursing home beds or from nursing home owners who fear a decline in profits. Take the example of the Harmar House Convalescent Home in Marietta, Ohio, where thirty-two patients died from asphyxiation in a fire in January, 1970. The home had been rated substandard on its fire and safety practices from 1967 to 1969. Shortly before the fire, the surveyor reported to the Social Security Administration that the home had removed these deficiencies though in fact deficiencies still existed. Medicare inspections were made by a county health department nurse. One of Harmar House's principal owners is the county coroner, whose wife is the city health officer of Marietta. Other owners include some of the most prominent physicians and businessmen in the community.* It is unreasonable to assume that all local inspectors use their discretion to uphold high standards when faced with implied or exercised pressure from nursing home owners who are also their neighbors and sometimes their bosses.

Nursing home inspections are often less revealing than they might be because of the almost universal practice of notifying the homes well in advance of the exact day and hour of the inspection. Thus the home has ample opportunity to disguise defects for the duration of the day's inspection. One of our correspondents reported a home that hired more personnel for the inspection day so that it would qualify under the staffing requirements. Another correspondent wrote that a home moved staff from floor to floor as the inspector made his tour, so that the proper number of nurses, aides, orderlies, etc., would be present on each floor. "Why does the Board of Health give advance notice of inspection?" the letter writer wanted to know. "They work like beavers for that one day. If you watched one of these [inspections] you would find it very amusing, but sickening."

Two members of this study visited a nursing home in Washington with a man who had spoken to us before of the smell and filth there. He was stunned to find the home clean the day of our visit. About three weeks later, he called to say he had discovered that the home had been preparing for an announced inspection. He reiterated his amazement on seeing the home so clean, repeating that he had never seen it so clean before or after that visit.

The failure of Federal authorities to enforce standards—indeed the Federal government's encouragement at the beginning of the Medicare program to waive

---

* See Chapter 3, Section 2 for a full discussion of the Harmar House fire.

standards—set the tone of laxity that has persisted at state and local levels. The argument of expediency is rarely a sound one in the long run, especially when it affects the lives and health and happiness of one million elderly Americans.

The Social Security Administration should act to remove the category of substantial compliance from its certification procedures and give notice to substandard homes that they will have to comply within a specific period of time.

The SSA, or any agency that assumes the total responsibility for nursing home care, should make public its ratings of individual institutions. At present, the Medicare "brand" may reassure the elderly and their families that they will receive adequate care in a particular home, although the facility actually falls below the requirements. Ratings should be coordinated with the level of care offered by the institution but should not fall below the level necessary for the well-being of any elderly person.

Finally, the Social Security Administration should assume its rightful responsibility by providing explicit instruction for the closing or decertification of substandard nursing homes.

MEDICAID AND THE NURSING HOME

The Federal government also became involved with nursing homes through Medicaid, Title XIX of the Social Security Act, which broadened the range of health services provided to people receiving Old Age Assistance payments and to the "medically indigent" receiving medical "vendors" payments under the Kerr-Mills Act of 1960. The new benefits include assistance payments for care in nursing homes. The administrative agency for Medicaid is the Medical Services Administration (MSA) of the Social and Rehabilitation Services of HEW, since it is a public assistance program. This means, however, that Medicaid standards for nursing homes are not coordinated with those applied under Medicare by the Social Security Administration. The SSA labels its nursing homes Extended Care Facilities while the MSA refers to "skilled nursing homes." The difference is not defined and often homes are certified under both programs, but under different standards.

Initially there was little reason for coordination of standards; the MSA definition of skilled nursing homes, issued in March, 1967, was so minimal there were, in effect, no standards. The rationale was that since Medicaid was to be administered by the states, the states should be responsible for protecting the interests of patients in nursing homes. By 1967, however, following the hearings by the Senate Committee on Aging that revealed the inadequacy of state licensing standards, Congressional concern arose over the quality of nursing home care.

Senators Frank Moss of Utah, Edward Kennedy of Massachusetts, and others, recognized the need for Federal standards to upgrade the nursing homes receiving Federal funds under Medicaid. (Some twelve thousand nursing homes receive Medicaid funds, three times the number of homes certified for Medicare.) The Moss amendments to Title XIX of the Social Security Act, passed in 1967, include disclosure of 10 per cent or more ownership of nursing homes; better standards in nursing homes, particularly those dealing with staffing requirements; and medical review. The Kennedy amendment calls for licensing of nursing home administrators.* The amendments were signed into law on January 2, 1968, but the regulations to implement the law and provide nursing home standards were not published until April 29, 1970. At the root of this classic instance of bureaucratic delay was Dr. Francis L. Land, then Commissioner of the Medical Services Administration.

It was Dr. Land's responsibility to draw up regulations for nursing homes receiving Federal funds. It was to be expected that pressure from nursing home owners would immediately be applied to keep the regulations minimal, but Dr. Land allowed these pressures to frustrate the adoption of regulations for two years, during which

* See Chapter 3, Section 4, for a complete discussion of the fate of this amendment.

time he appointed or reappointed numerous groups which prepared some fifteen different drafts of regulations.

The argument of the nursing home industry was that if standards were too high, no nursing home would qualify for Medicaid, thereby making the program no more than an "academic benefit" which looked good on paper but could not be implemented.[24] Other people, including the AFL-CIO and the National Council of Senior Citizens, urged establishment of tight standards at the beginning, pointing to the difficulties under the Medicare program of forcing homes to upgrade standards once they were certified.

Senator Moss finally intervened, questioned the delay, and held hearings on the regulations on July 31, 1969. At the hearings, William R. Hutton, representing the National Council of Senior Citizens, denounced the interim regulations published by MSA in June, 1969, saying that when compared to the intent of the Moss amendments of 1967, "the interests of the nursing home industry have been accommodated and the aged have been sold short." [25]

Dr. Land did not appear at the hearings; he had resigned the day before.

After the hearings and Dr. Land's resignation, a new task force was appointed to review the drafts of regulations that had been proposed. The task force made a series of recommendations that in effect urged adoption of the first draft, drawn up early in January, 1969. On April 29, 1970, these regulations were finally published in the *Federal Register*.

Although the regulations were at last in effect, it was still left to the states to implement them. The MSA proved even less capable than the Social Security Administration in overseeing the process of inspection. When Medicaid was enacted in 1965, the entire Medical Services Administration had a staff of eighty-four people. They were to administer a program that by January, 1968, with thirty-seven states participating, was costing 3.54 billion dollars.[26] Yet it was not until a reorganization of MSA in May, 1970, that its staff grew from eighty-four to 156 employees.

The manpower problem of the nursing home part of the program has reached critical proportions. Nursing home benefits under Medicaid currently involve Federal and state expenditures of 1.2 billion dollars to some twelve thousand nursing homes. The function of the MSA nursing home branch is to develop standards for skilled nursing homes, implement the 1967 amendments, and assist the states through consultation. The MSA nursing home branch has grown from one to four staff members since the program began. One official estimates that it needs from sixteen to eighteen staff members to implement the program adequately. No matter how high the standards, it is not likely that four Federal employees can make a great impact on their implementation in nursing homes across the nation.

MSA officials admit that there is no effort within the agency to enforce standards in Medicaid homes. Regional offices, where the focus of enforcement might logically rest, have an average of four employees. By default, officials say, the only enforcement efforts now stem from the General Accounting Office, "the government's F.B.I.," which audits Medicaid and other Federal programs to see that money is not squandered.

If anything is clear in the bureaucratic haze that engulfs Federal involvement with nursing homes today, it is that the elderly patient is denied assurance of proper care and a decent home.

3 Inside the Nursing Home

THE JOURNALS

June 26. FORGET IT! I AM NEVER GOING BACK!

June 27. That was written last night, just after I returned from my first night at the *** home. What is really bad is that instead of coming up with a crusader wish to help the nursing home problem, I came out last night vowing to commit suicide before I get old. (Claire Townsend)

June 27. The head nurse or supervisor, a licensed practical nurse, told us that she was glad we had come because usually she had only three people to work her intensive care floor of about fifty-four patients. (Elizabeth Baldwin)

June 27. In one home we went to, an aide with no experience was left alone on her second night to prepare twenty bedridden patients for bed. One woman expressed a desire to get out of bed and go to the toilet. The aide, having never actually gotten a patient out of bed, just watched it done once, got the woman into the bathroom, supporting most of the woman's weight, and onto the toilet seat. When the patient was done, the aide walked her back to bed, but as the bed was a high hospital type, the aide was not strong enough to lift the woman in and ended up rolling her onto it with much pain and consternation to both. (Janet Keyes)

June 27. I followed one nurse around today and asked her to explain what she was doing—like the tests for sugar and acid in the urine. When the former came out negative, I asked her if that was good and she said, "No . . . yes . . . no . . . wait a minute . . . yes, it's good to be negative, but not too negative."

The nurse I was assigned to, Grace, was so kind to some patients and so mean to others that it was cruel when the two extremes happened in a single room with two patients. While the two of us were putting the favored patient to bed (doing a lot of extra fussing and smiling and taking a long time) the other patient kept saying, "Girlie, please put me to bed." But I did not know how to go about it, so I just stood there feeling helpless and horrible. Then Grace finally ambled over to the second patient, jerked her out of the chair, slammed her against the bed, and roughly undressed her. The patient kept crying and saying that she was about to slip and fall, but Grace just told her to shut up. Finally, I assisted the woman up onto the bed. Then Grace threw the covers over her, covering her face, so I had to uncover her and tuck her in. (Claire Townsend)

July 4. The Colonel tried to tip me twenty-five cents for taking him to the bathroom. (Patricia Pittis)

June 27. When it came time to give the medicine, the R.N. said she was too busy, and would we please administer it. Later, Grace told me what we had just done was illegal, that only an R.N. can administer medicine. (Claire Townsend)

July 1. The aide called all the old people "the little people who do crazy things" and said you can never trust them, because they never take their medicine or do what they are supposed to do.

Schedule for the day shift, 7:00 A.M. to 3:00 P.M. Fourteen people to take care of—seven per aide. All on different floors and all to be waked at different hours. I would go into their rooms with Mrs. B.'s master key, wake them up, wash them down with a brief sponge bath, take them to the bathroom, partially dress them (shoes and dressing gown), and open their breakfast for them if it had already arrived.

Breakfast generally consisted of some form of eggs with cold toast and jam, coffee, milk or orange juice. (Patricia Pittis)

June 28. On the lunch tray there were two dry fish sticks, some mashed potatoes, and puréed peas (everyone gets the puréed food whether or not they are on a special diet), and some cornbread. As one tray was being carried down the hall to a patient, a nurse reached over, picked up a piece of cornbread from the tray, and ate it. (Claire Townsend)

July 3. All they ever do is watch TV, eat, and sleep. Some do not even care what they watch—they are not listening anyway. They just sit in their chairs and stare blankly at the noise coming out of the TV. Although the *** home schedules trips regularly (recently went to see the Hershey chocolate factory in Pennsylvania), bingo twice a week, movies on Fridays, birthday parties once a month, religious services on Thursdays and Sundays, all of this does not seem to fill up the time, and few seem to participate. (Patricia Pittis)

June 28. A no-legged man died at 9:00 A.M. the morning of my second day; they did not get his body removed until 11:00 that night. The R.N. said she had called the doctor to come over to pronounce him dead (that was what they were waiting for all the time), but he never came. Finally the friendly neighborhood mortician picked up the body and drove it to the hospital where a doctor could be found. (Claire Townsend)

July 13. Mrs. M. is totally incontinent. Came in to put her to bed and found her already in her nightgown. She had not been dressed all day. Her nightgown was soaked. Her urine had run down her legs, through her stockings, and into her shoes, which were now soaked also. No one had done anything for her or checked her since she had been gotten up around 8:30 A.M. She should have gone downstairs long ago, but she hated to disturb the nurses—she knows they are so busy. All she does is sit in her urine-soaked clothing all day, watching television, but not really concentrating. (Patricia Pittis)

June 28. It got so it seemed that all we did for eight

hours was clean up crap and empty urine bags. (Claire Townsend)

June 27. The air conditioning got the rooms much too cold and could not be turned off. Most of the patients were shivering and I was shivering, too. When we came on the morning round there were not enough blankets for everybody. (Elizabeth Baldwin)

July 1. Some rooms smelled atrocious because of little or no ventilation. Some patients had air conditioning; others could not open their windows. Still others said they would be cold if we opened their windows for them. (Patricia Pittis)

June 27. The fingernails and toenails of the patients were long and disgustingly dirty. (Elizabeth Baldwin)

July 2. There does not seem to be any rehabilitation program. One man, totally bedridden, never even wore any clothes. He sat up to eat, then went right back to bed. Mr. T. is ambulatory with a cane and walker, but we took him down to the taxi in a wheelchair because "it was faster and more convenient," according to Mrs. B. Mrs. B. said there was a whirlpool in the basement, but did not say how often it was used, or by whom. (Patricia Pittis)

July 6. The physical therapist is supposed to come in every Tuesday but sometimes he never comes. (Patricia Pittis)

June 27. Mrs. W. was a big black woman in her fifties or sixties who kept saying she was burning "down there." It turned out that her skin had been split open as a result of aides' carelessness in turning her over. This had happened before and she had been hospitalized as a result. This time all they put on it was a towel.

Another lady had a catheter tube without a urinal bag attached to it. (Elizabeth Baldwin)

July 2. There are no regular fire drills and Mrs. B. said that patients have no idea what they are supposed to do in case of fire. When some kids came in and pulled the alarm for fun, all the ambulatory patients stood in the halls and wondered what was going on, and where the fire was. It would be a mad house if a fire were to occur. None of the aides or most of the staff have any idea of the best way to evacuate the building; as far as I can see, there is no organized plan. The nearest available exits are not posted anywhere. (Patricia Pittis)

June 27. One thing that surprised me was that patients were allowed to smoke in bed at night, a serious fire hazard. (Elizabeth Baldwin)

June 27. The nurses were all smoking, so I asked in which rooms was smoking permissible. "Nowhere. But we sneak cigarettes in here and in the lounge all the time. It don't make no difference." Half the time I see the R.N. smoking as she walks down the hall. (Claire Townsend)

July 2. Personal records of health are kept. Drugs administered to patients are recorded on same sheet with date. Also each shift writes down what happened during their shift. If anyone fell, died, got sick, sent to the hospital, or went home or away. (Patricia Pittis)

June 27. One lady, one of the few who could talk sensibly, said that the doctor comes in, just asks her how she feels, and then leaves, charging her ten dollars. (Elizabeth Baldwin)

July 6. According to Mrs. B., there are three doctors at the *** home. Two doctors charge ten dollars per patient per visit, even if it takes place in the office, while the third tells them to leave what they can afford on her desk when they go out. The patients leave two to three dollars, which does not even pay for the shots they are given, much less the doctor's visit. Therefore, it is understandable that she has the most patients in the nursing home. The doctor has reserved Tuesdays and Thursdays for visits, from 10:00 A.M. to 2:00 P.M. Mrs. B. says she never gets a chance to see all her patients during those two days, so some go for two weeks or more without being able to see their doctor. (Patricia Pittis)

July 10. Mrs. C. fell during the night. She has lacerations all up her right arm. Her left arm has been put in a cast. The blood on her wounds has already dried and crusted around the edges. It must have been a long time before she called the nursing station to ask for help. When we arrived, the room stank; the bathroom floor,

sink, and tub, and the bedroom carpet were covered
with blood and feces—Mrs. C. and her bed, too. Beth
gave her a quick bath and took her blood pressure;
I changed her bed. Both of us were nurses' aides and
did not know what else to do. Nurse S. was scheduled
to come in that morning but she never showed up—
did not call to give an explanation or anything. In fact,
when we called her, the phone was disconnected. She
had not come in all week. . . . We were not authorized
to give medication. At 8:30 we called Mrs. R. when the
nurse was still not in. She was furious at us for not telling her sooner. . . . Meanwhile, the diabetic patients
had to be given their insulin at the exact time. So a
private nurse gave it to them while I took care of her
patient. Finally, Mrs. B. came in; she was supposed to
be on vacation.

I saw the whole list of applications and changes of
personnel. Beth plans to leave; Martha plans to leave
eventually; I plan to leave before the end of the summer.
Nurse S. never comes in anyway, so there will be no one
left in the nursing station in a few weeks.

The conditions are too bad to stay long. Already I am
feeling less cheerful, I am less patient and rougher with
the patients. They get me down. I begin to think and
feel like them with all their pains! (Patricia Pittis)

July 11. Beth took money out of the Colonel's coat
pocket when she thought I could not see her. But I saw
her doing it in the mirror. She is very underhanded and
suspicious; she looked guiltily back to see if I were there
every few seconds, then took the money. I was in the
bathroom helping the Colonel go to the bathroom.
(Patricia Pittis)

June 27. I heard one of the nurses ask another nurse,
"Do you have Mrs. B.'s cold cream?" And the other
nurse said, "No, E. has Mrs. B.'s cold cream. But I have
her hand lotion." (Claire Townsend)

July 11. Mrs. B. came in in the morning and found a
plastic jar that had contained a thousand aspirins completely empty. She did not know who had taken
them but thought maybe the kitchen help and other employees had asked for them until there were none left.

She did not make a big fuss about the issue. (Patricia Pittis)

July 12. All the old people have to look forward to is meals—it is one of the only events in their entire daily routine. There are three different servings for dinner: 4:15, 5:15, 6:15. Exactly on the dot they all rush to the door and stampede in like little children in school starving for their lunch. They sit on the sofas and chairs in the hallway up to forty-five minutes or an hour waiting for their mealtime to roll around. Others wait up to an hour in the theater in the front seats waiting for the movie at 7:00 P.M. There is nothing else to look forward to, I guess. (Patricia Pittis)

June 27. We sat around the nursing station at 12:20 A.M., talking and playing the radio, drinking water and coffee and eating pizza for about half an hour—right across the hall from a patient's room whose door was open. (Elizabeth Baldwin)

July 11. Mrs. R. told me that the only way to get the hospital to send out an ambulance to pick up the Colonel for his checkup would be if he were lying on the floor of his room. When Beth and I took him to the bathroom, he happened to lose his footing, so Beth casually let him drop to the floor of the bathroom and then called Mrs. B. The ambulance men were angry because the manager had lied and told the hospital that the Colonel had had a heart attack. The hospital gave him a quick checkup, but the Colonel says they did not ask him a thing. They sent him back right away.

The man in room 165 is so lonely. He wants a nurse in there every minute of the day and does not let you go until he knows exactly when you will be back and who the nurse is on the next shift, if you will not be back until the next day. I asked him how his dinner had been, and he said, "Never very good and always lonely." (Patricia Pittis)

June 27. In the *** home, there were almost no activities. On warm days, the patients were wheeled up to the front porch where they were able to watch the cars rush by on a dirty highway, or overlook the adjacent cemetery. A few watched an unfocused television, while others sat around the nurses' station and stared absently at the opening and shutting of the elevator door. There were no newspapers, magazines, or books in evidence and rarely any planned activities. Once a week, a cart was brought around from the local drugstore and the patients were able to pay exorbitant prices to buy a few items to brighten up their day. Immediately after dinner, the patients started asking the nurses if they could go to bed; they had nothing else to do. (Janet Keyes)

FIRE IN OHIO

On January 9, 1970, thirty-two elderly patients died of smoke asphyxiation at a Marietta, Ohio, nursing home called the Harmar House Convalescent Home. The fire was put out in less than half an hour, but in the meantime, thick clouds of black smoke had filled the rooms and corridors of the home, suffocating twenty-one of the forty-six patients almost immediately. Eleven others died soon after. Not one of the dead had burned flesh. Most of the patients were in their late seventies or eighties; most were bedfast. The incident shocked the public and inquiries began almost immediately.

Investigations concluded that a cigarette was the immediate cause of the fire.[1] Officials guessed that it began when the elderly occupant of room 104, or an employee, dropped a lighted cigarette or emptied an ashtray into a plastic wastebasket. Fire spread from the basket to a wooden night stand and a plastic-covered chair as well as to the carpet of the room. A heat sensor in the room alerted the nursing station when the temperature hit 136 degrees Fahrenheit. Two of the home's four employees on that shift, an aide and a practical nurse, answered the alarm in room 104 and found dense smoke billowing from the room. The aide, a nineteen-year-old girl weighing eighty-seven pounds, made it into the room and carried the resident to safety. She did not close the door of the room behind her. Smoke was by now filling the corridor. The employees began moving patients outside. Someone left the corridor door open and other wings began to fill with smoke.

The Marietta fire chief estimated that there had been a four-minute delay before the bewildered staff telephoned the fire department. The aide who had discovered the fire said later that she thought the heat sensor signaled the fire department automatically, which it did not. Firemen arrived within five minutes and the fire was out within twelve minutes.

It was not long before the fire shifted to the Social Security Administration, which had certified Harmar House as a Medicare home. The investigations that followed disillusioned those who believed that the Medicare stamp meant safety. It also revealed that even under unusual pressure to act on a question of safety, the Social Security Administration seemed unable to do so with clarity and dispatch. The particular question posed by the Harmar House fire was whether the SSA would act decisively to remove unsafe carpeting from nursing homes. Eight months after the fire, the SSA invited public comment on proposed standards for new carpet, but as of January, 1971, no standards were in effect. SSA has never even proposed standards for already existing carpet. Thus, the larger question is whether the SSA is providing decisive leadership to insure safety in other areas of the nursing home, and whether questions of safety should be referred to the Social Security Administration in the first place.

Harmar House was a classic example of the breakdown in standard enforcement. From 1967 to 1969, the home was listed as deficient in "specifications of alarm signals, frequency of fire drills, and assignment of personnel responsibility in a crisis." [2] In April, 1969, the county health department nurse surveying the facility reported that the deficiencies had been removed; apparently they had not been. At the time of the fire, Harmar House had had no fire drill in ten months, although Medicare standards require a drill at least three times a year. Employees testified that they had no idea what their duties were in case of an emergency. The aide who rescued the patient in room 104 had been working at the home for several months but had never been told that one of the first principles of confining fire is to close the door of the room where the fire starts. The four-minute delay in notifying the fire department was due in part to her mistaken belief that the room sensor automatically signaled the fire department.

Investigators began to go farther. There were no fire doors in the 244-foot north-south corridor. Hill-Burton and the Life Safety Code of the National Fire Protection Association call for at least one division every 150 feet of corridor. The state code was ambiguous, but Medicare relied on state and local codes.[3]

According to one report, the door to room 104 was too narrow to admit a hospital bed. Even if true, it was not in violation of state or Medicare regulations. Medicare regulations left widths of doorways, corridors, and aisles to the discretion of the surveyors, saying only that they should be "wide enough for easy evacuation."[4] In addition, the home had no sprinklers; none were required.[5]

Local officials were quick to put the blame on the SSA for leaving important safety measures to the discretion of local inspectors. Marietta Mayor John A. Brunworth told the Moss committee, "One responsibility the federal government has is to do things for us we can't do for ourselves. I'm not against federal intervention if it's for the benefit of the patient."[6]

W. H. Veigel of the Ohio Department of Health also told a reporter: "As a person reviewing surveys, I think it is time Medicare people showed some intestinal fortitude by letting operators of nursing homes know what's important." He termed the Medicare and the Ohio code "weak."[7]

Beyond the general inadequacy of safety standards, the particular villain in the Harmar House fire was the carpet, whose foam-rubber backing caused the smoke that killed the thirty-two patients. The Ohio code allows carpeting that has a flame spread rating of up to 200 when tested by the tunnel test.* The carpet in Harmar House had a flame spread of 275. Ohio authorities said they were never informed that the carpet had been installed, nor was there any report of its flame

___

* For explanations of the flammability tests, see note 9, page 179.

spread characteristics to the state before the fire. Although state building inspectors had visited the home, none apparently had asked about the carpet.[8]

Medicare had simply incorporated the state standards for carpeting by reference. Both the Life Safety Code and the Hill-Burton construction standards for hospitals and nursing homes built with Federal grants recommend that interior finishes, such as carpeting, have no more than a 75 flame spread rating. The carpet in the Harmar House had almost four times the flame spread potential considered safe for institutions by Federal safety authorities.

The first action on the part of the government came ten days after the fire, when the Public Health Service circulated a memorandum to state agencies advising against the use of carpet and carpet assemblies with flame spread ratings of more than 75.

On February 9, Chairman Moss of the Senate Subcommittee on Long-Term Care opened hearings on the fire. The SSA had still not drafted proposals for new carpeting regulations, and Senator Moss urged them to close this gap in the regulations rapidly. At the same hearing, Jack Bono of Underwriters' Laboratories, Inc., presented his organization's findings on three flammability tests performed on the Harmar House carpet at the request of the Ohio fire marshal.[9]

The tests were the methenamine pill test, the Steiner tunnel test, and a chamber test recently developed by U.L. The carpet would have "passed" the pill test and failed both the tunnel and chamber tests. The assessment of these three tests, and the pressure of the carpet industry for the adoption of the relatively weak pill test, delayed the SSA from proposing regulations until eight months after the fire.

Later in February, 1970, the Social Security Administration's Bureau of Health Insurance (BHI) sent out a vague memorandum instructing state agencies to forbid new installations of carpeting with a flame spread rating higher than 75. On already installed carpeting, the memo asked the Extended Care Facilities to find out the rating. If the rating were unknown or excessive, the state agency should ask the facility to explain the steps it would take to correct the deficiency or alternative steps to protect the environment from fire hazard; get a state or local fire authority to evaluate the steps; forward the findings to the BHI regional office for final decision.

One official mentioned sprinklers as an "alternative step," although the Public Health Service experts assert that they are not sufficient protection against rapid flame spread. (Carpet fires may generate a great deal of lethal smoke without generating enough heat to activate the sprinkler system.) The use of so-called flame-proofing was also suggested, though flame-proofing is generally regarded as insufficient because it is temporary and easily washes out.

The memo brought another flurry of criticism. Congressman David Pryor asked, "Eventually these standards [on carpet safety] must be issued. Why not now? If the Bureau of Health Insurance cannot act now when the terrible deaths of 32 helpless people are fresh in our minds, when will it act?" Another fact that struck Pryor as incredible was that two HEW programs—Hill-Burton and Medicare—lacked comparable safety standards for the same type of facility. In addition, in 1967, Congress made the Life Safety Code provisions applicable to Medicaid homes as of January 1, 1970. This left local surveyors in a quandary about homes that participated in both Medicare and Medicaid, as was the case with Harmar House. Finally, as of July 1, 1970, nursing homes are required to comply with whichever of the two standards (Medicare or Medicaid) is higher. Some states have adopted Medicaid standards that are considerably higher than Federal Medicare standards. It remains to be seen how this will be enforced in practice, and the basic question—why have two sets of standards in the first place?—remains unanswered.

Still the SSA was silent. According to officials, they were busy holding advisory sessions during the months after the hearing to determine the proper test to be used for carpets.[10] They talked, for example, with industry people about the development of a "new" flame-retardant spray. They discussed the pros and cons of the pill test with carpeting manufacturers, as well as with the Bureau of Standards. They waited for the National Fire Protection Association to make its own endorsement. (The NFPA eventually came out for the tunnel test.) They awaited word from Underwriters' Laboratories about progress on the chamber test to see whether they could incorporate that standard in their regulations.

An insight into the quandary at HEW and SSA may have been provided during a Moss subcommittee hearing in May, 1970. Val Halamanderis, staff investigator, asked SSA's Morris Levy the question he felt SSA was asking itself: "What kind of a standard are we [the SSA] going to issue, the situation being that we are caught in the middle—on the one hand, industry is on our necks and on the other hand, myself and Senator Moss. So we put our finger to the wind and determine which way the wind blows the hardest and we determine a standard."

On May 6, 1970, the Community Health Service of the Public Health Service, one of the advisory bodies to the SSA, endorsed the tunnel test as the only acceptable test method for carpeting available at that time.[11] In effect, the endorsement established the official HEW position. It had been cleared with top officials, and Mrs. Virginia Knauer, the President's advisor on consumer affairs, concurred.

Two months later, another memo issued from the office of Dr. Harold Graning of the Public Health Service, Health Facilities Planning and Construction Service (Hill-Burton), saying that carpeting that passed either the tunnel test or the chamber test should be acceptable for new installations. The memo rejected the pill test as ineffective and acknowledged the well-known criticisms of the tunnel test—that it "subjected materials to test conditions that were not similar to real life situations." Graning said that U.L. had finished studies of the chamber test; after careful consideration of the U.L. reports, his office "will be recommending to the Federal Hospital Council adoption of regulations in which the chamber test as devised by Underwriters' Laboratories will become the official test to be utilized for any carpeting that is to be used in any patient areas." [12]

The Graning memo added that "existing carpeting whose flammability is not known could be given the option of either being subjected to the chamber test or treated with flame-retardant sprays that are now available on the commercial market." [13] This latter option is not mentioned in any later memos or specifically mentioned in the proposed regulations.

In the midst of this debate over appropriate tests, the carpet industry was making a last-ditch plea for the pill test as the standard for all carpets and rugs. George Paules, President of the Carpet and Rug Institute, speaking before the Senate Subcommittee on the Consumer in June, attempted to discredit the tunnel test as "non-applicable" to carpeting and plugged the pill test as "a valid test for carpet." [14] He later tried to discredit the tunnel and chamber tests by calling them "ridiculous." He dismissed the concern of safety and health officials, saying that their adopted tests "satisfied an emotional rather than a purposeful need." [15] Paules also suggested to the Committee that the Harmar House tragedy could have been prevented by sprinklers, although fire safety experts testified that even if Harmar House had had a fire sprinkler system it would have not been effective because of the speed at which the fire had progressed.[16]

The pill test had been adopted by the Department of Commerce on April 13, 1970, as the national standard for carpeting used in homes, offices, restaurants, etc. But the Public Health Service found the test "not designed specifically to provide the degree of protection necessary for institutional type occupancy where the occupants are not freely ambulatory, such as a nursing home, hospital, or home "for the aged." [17] The Bureau of Standards itself admits that the pill test was developed as a "quick and dirty test" and that currently much work is being done to make the test more definitive.[18]

One reason for the carpet industry's vigorous advocacy of the pill test, and attempt to discredit the tunnel test, was suggested in a report to the National Commission on Product Safety by David Apter and Associates:

> While responding in a public-spirited manner to develop the standard, the carpet and rug industry would like to offset the inroads made by the Hill-Burton standards [the

tunnel test] of the Department of Health, Education and Welfare, lest the Hill-Burton standards or some other rigorous standard set the requirements for all carpets and rugs, particularly those used in institutions such as schools and public buildings.[19]

It is to the credit of the SSA that it has not yet succumbed to the urgings of the carpet industry. When its proposed regulations were finally made public in the *Federal Register* on September 2, 1970—eight months less a week after the disastrous fire in Marietta, Ohio— they included the Life Safety Code, use of the tunnel test with a rating of 75 in patient areas of the nursing home, or use of the chamber test. The SSA rejected the weaker pill test.

A major question that still remained unanswered is whether the SSA is qualified to set safety standards, or whether that responsibility should rest with the Public Health Service staff of safety experts who developed the carpeting standards for Hill-Burton programs in 1965. Although they had been consulted in drawing up the Medicare Extended Care Facility regulations in 1966, carpeting was not mentioned in the initial SSA regulations. The confusion over which test is appropriate for carpets in nursing homes appears sufficiently serious to warrant a decision by safety experts; the SSA, however, has no safety experts on its staff.

A further problem is that after taking eight months even to suggest standards to cover newly installed carpet, the SSA has not yet promulgated guidelines for homes that already have carpeting—by far the vast majority. The best of tests will have little meaning if it is not applied to nursing homes which may already have hazardous carpeting. When asked about this, BHI officials were vague. They are "struggling with" this question as of this writing, according to one official.[20] The office is trying to determine whether it is feasible to retain unsafe carpeting if other "appropriate safeguards" are taken. However, as in the early stages of the controversy, officials are still unable to define exactly what is meant by "adequate alternative" to removal of unsafe carpeting. The possibilities are to demand that the carpet be taken out immediately; to let the carpeting remain in the institution so that the home can receive a five-year write-off for tax purposes; or to allow a faster tax write-off for Medicare purposes. According to one official, criteria are being devised which would allow unsafe carpeting to remain in the home until the tax write-off period ends.

Shortage of testing facilities for carpet flammability is one reason given for developing "alternative criteria" that would, in effect, allow a home to waive the test and retain its untested carpeting.[21] However, Underwriters' Laboratories has made available to the Bureau of Standards instructions for test construction. It is not reassuring that instead of taking steps to construct testing facilities, the SSA is instead developing "alternative criteria."

Finally, the proposed regulations make a distinction between "nonpatient" areas of nursing homes, and "patient" areas, where carpets must meet more stringent tests. Morris Levy of the Bureau of Health Insurance, Division of State Operations, said his office will be issuing instructions to states as to precisely how this distinction is to be made. For example, the patient area will include the areas in which "most of the patient's time is spent": his room, the adjacent corridors, recreational areas, etc.[22] The patient area must also have doors that will close it off from the rest of the nursing home where more flammable carpet may be installed. Once again a question arises: Is it wise to have carpeting anywhere in a nursing home where some risks may be involved?

A year after the Marietta fire, SSA still lacked a regulation to require the removal of dangerous carpeting from facilities, even following the unusual public and political pressure caused by the widely publicized tragedy in Ohio. Although SSA had prevented—without regulation—*installations* of carpeting that would not meet the Hill-Burton standard, SSA said it could not require *removal* unless it had a regulation. How soon a regulation would be written and go into effect—with or without the tunnel test—was unclear even as late as February, 1971. If SSA, as was indicated, decided to accept the chamber test, then again HEW would have a divided policy: Medicare, pulling Medicaid along with it, would drop the tunnel test but Hill-Burton would keep it. The implications reach beyond the question of carpeting, which is only one safety factor in nursing homes. Instead of acting with clarity and dispatch to remove a clear hazard from all nursing homes, the SSA responded with confusion and delay. On the issue of new carpet tests, its responsibility for the safety of nursing home residents was not matched by the expertise to make judgments about safety. On the issue of the safety of existing carpet, the agency's concern for the costs to nursing home operators has been allowed to delay action on existing hazards. Will the SSA demand alarm signals, fire drills, disaster plan instructions, and fire doors for nursing homes? There is no indication that homes lacking these basic safety precautions will not continue to be approved under "substantial" compliance. Nor is there evidence that the SSA plans to make sure that homes like Harmar House—which had been listed as having corrected fire safety deficiencies—really have accomplished what inspectors say they have. The larger issue for nursing homes is that when the SSA had the opportunity to take a clear stand for strong enforcement, it failed to do so. In May SSA's Levy said there were "something like a thousand facilities with carpeting that does not meet the tunnel test" and many that had yet to learn what the flame spreads were of their carpeting. As this was written, for all SSA knew, thousands of patients remained in jeopardy, and had remained so during the year and longer since Marietta.

DEATH IN MARYLAND

The twenty-year-old manager of a Fairfax County pet store that advertises "instant credit—pay as you love" was convicted of two counts of cruelty to animals yesterday and fined one thousand dollars with all but two hundred dollars suspended.

Ruling that the care and treatment of animals is a matter of common sense, Fairfax County Court Judge J. Mason Grove rejected a defense lawyer's argument that the county lacks established pet store standards that would prevent the humane society from "coming down and getting [an arrest] warrant any time they want."

The judge fined the manager, Norman Leppert, five hundred dollars on each of two charges and suspended

eight hundred dollars of the fines on the condition that
Leppert steers clear of future violations.

The charges against Leppert alleged that on July 16
and 17 he failed to treat humanely several dogs for sale
at the Docktor Pet Center, 7263 Arlington Blvd.

Another allegation was that Leppert was warned on a
Monday that a Norwegian elkhound was ill but did not
summon a veterinarian until the following Friday.[1]

On Friday, July 31, 1970, Dr. Neil Solomon, Secretary
of Health and Mental Hygiene for Maryland, received
a report that nine residents of the Gould Convalesarium
in Baltimore had died of salmonella poisoning.[2] Salmonella is a family of bacteria that can cause an infectious
disease marked by nausea, diarrhea, and dehydration,
and can be particularly serious to the elderly and the
very young.

The first outbreak of the epidemic was apparent on
Monday, July 27, four days before state health authorities were notified. The first victim was not hospitalized
until Friday, July 31, by which time ninety-five of the
home's 144 residents had shown symptoms of the disease
and eleven had died. The last of the twenty-five deaths
that were attributed to salmonella poisoning occurred
August 23. Between July 26, when the meal suspected
as the cause was served, and August 23, 108 of the
residents showed symptoms of salmonella poisoning.

According to testimony at hearings on August 19
before the Senate Subcommittee on Long-Term Care,
this incident reached epidemic proportions with a 28
per cent mortality rate and 70 per cent of the population
at the Convalesarium showing symptoms. Thirty of the
seventy-six employees showed signs of the disease as
well.[3]

It was also revealed at the hearings that the Gould
Convalesarium did not meet state requirements for
kitchen hygiene or food distribution. The rinse water
for dishes was not considered hot enough and the institution was criticized by health surveyors for improper
food handling.[4]

The meal apparently containing the lethal bacteria
was served at supper on Sunday, July 26, and consisted
of deviled eggs and shrimp salad. Although the exact

cause was not determined, witnesses at the August hearings of the Subcommittee said that either the eggs were cracked or the prepared food had been permitted to sit out with no refrigeration for too long, or that someone handling the food carried the germs.

The conditions that allowed the epidemic to occur in the first place raised the old question of inspections and enforcement of sanitation standards. Mrs. Ruth Murphy, a Medicare coordinator for the state health department, told a panel appointed by the Maryland Secretary of Health and Mental Hygiene that her review of health department records indicated that nursing home inspections had been haphazardly carried out.[5] Some inspectors, she said, overlooked unsanitary conditions or questionable food practices.

Mrs. Murphy also said she had discovered inconsistencies in inspection reports. "Everything is checked right, indicating everything is right in the [nursing] home and then you get a lot of complaints from the public indicating otherwise," she testified.[6]

Thus, the initial problem—the fact that such an outbreak could occur—could be traced in part to the lack of rigid inspections. This was true despite the fact that city and state authorities gave the Gould home good marks. All witnesses said it was as good or better than its competitors and that sanitary conditions were "satisfactory"—a word that the *Post* reporter noted was often used during the course of the panel's hearings.

A major concern of the panel was the delay in reporting the epidemic to state health officials. It seemed that no one—neither the administration, nor the nursing staff, nor the doctors who treated patients at the home— took it upon himself to report it initially. Dr. John V. DeHoff, then acting city health commissioner for Baltimore, testified that had the epidemic been reported earlier, some of the deaths might have been prevented.[7] For two days, the panel tried to elicit an explanation for what it first took to be an extraordinary case of negligence. The picture that gradually emerged was not one of unusual or exceptional neglect but one of "customary" nursing home practice—no regular communication between physicians and nursing home staff, and no acceptance of responsibility by physicians for conditions in the home.

Sarah Hawkins, a state health official, was told of the outbreak during a routine visit but failed to report it to her superiors. She told a committee of the State Medical Society, which also investigated the incident, that she was not alarmed by what she learned. Furthermore, she was "under the pressure of filming a documentary on nursing homes" at the time.[8]

The failure to report the incident immediately was the second fundamental and frightening fact. Here, the investigating panel found a deeper problem that lay behind both the epidemic's occurrence and the failure to report it quickly—a lack of any medical supervision of medical conditions in the home as a whole.

Maryland's communicable disease law requires that when there are three or more cases of communicable disease, particularly food poisoning, the city health department must be notified immediately. There were forty-four physicians who treated patients at the home; some visited patients during the first four days of the epidemic before the report was made. Some apparently knew of the epidemic, but no one reported it. Doctors testified they did not necessarily confer with the staff during their visits to patients and had therefore received no "formal" report of an epidemic. Dr. Harold V. Harbold, the home's "principal physician," said that he was not "fully" aware of the extent of the disease since he treated only his own patients, and was not informed of the epidemic by the staff.

The owner of the home, Mitchell Gould, insisted to the investigating panel that doctors did know about the epidemic. Arnold M. Weiner, Gould's lawyer, said Harbold and other physicians had been kept informed by the staff and had even made references to the epidemic in their reports. When a *Post* reporter asked Harbold about this allegation, the doctor said he heard some "loose talk" about widespread diarrhea but added that he never was formally informed of the apparent epidemic. "I didn't know what was going on because there's no tie-in between the principal physician and the home," was Harbold's startling explanation to the *Post*.[9]

Dr. Harbold also told the panel that the term "principal physician" was meaningless in practice. The term meant only that he treated patients who had no other personal physician, he said. Dr. Harbold was treating thirty-nine patients at the time of the epidemic, eleven of whom died following the outbreak. Fifteen of his patients had diarrhea within the first two days of the outbreak. Harbold, whose fees are paid by the patients or through Medicare but not by Gould, said he did not report the outbreak of diarrhea to public health officials because he considered it common among the aged. Referring to the visit of Sarah Hawkins to the home during the outbreak, Harbold said he considered a visit by a state health official notice enough.

Also playing musical chairs with the question of responsibility was owner Mitchell Gould, whose remarkable explanation for the tragedy was that the epidemic was caused by the city's water supply. "We had a problem with water for quite some time," Gould told the panel. "The water had been dirty and murky. Solid particles had lodged in the toilets." [10] According to the *Post* report, a procession of health and sanitation experts said the likely cause was either shrimp salad or deviled eggs served at dinner on July 26. They said they could not be absolutely sure of their findings, but they distinctly ruled out the city's water supply. If the community's water had been at fault, the epidemic would have struck outside the nursing home, too.[11]

Undoubtedly several factors went into the making of the tragedy in Maryland. All of them—inaction on the part of public health officials, as well as lack of responsibility assumed within the home—were outlined in the report of the investigating panel, which was published in October, 1970. The role of the physicians in the incident illuminates an absence of direct medical responsibility in the nursing home that is particularly troubling. A committee of the State Medical and Chirurgical Faculty of the Maryland Medical Society investigated the incident and found that the attending physicians had violated two state laws by failing to report the epidemic immediately. The committee did not recommend any punishment.[12] The reasons for this recommendation, according to Dr. Matthew Tayback of the Maryland Health Department, were that no single physician could technically be held responsible for the total health care in the home; the medical society committee found nothing "malicious" in the failure of the doctors to make the report; and the committee found in their actions *"nothing contrary to usual medical practice."* [13] (Emphasis added.)

The Maryland Health Department is attempting to find a means of enforcing physicians' responsibility for the total medical care of a nursing home by formulating a new concept of "medical director." The medical director, Dr. Tayback said, would be clearly responsible for the medical care in a home; he would supervise policies for admission, see that patient care policies were carried out as stated, and supervise the medical aspects of hygiene. The medical director would not necessarily be a permanent staff member, but his responsibilities would be specifically outlined and carry the added incentive of extra pay.

The problem of enforcement is the major drawback to the concept of medical director. Simply adding specific duties to the "meaningless" title of "principal physician" will have little effect unless the state can insure that the duties are performed. As Dr. Tayback admitted, physicians object strenuously to any hint of interference in their treatment of patients, either by external authorities or by colleagues. Nursing home operators may object if dictates by the medical director lead to costly improvements in the nursing home. If the operator objects and the medical director does not insist—perhaps because he does not wish to lose the supplementary income from the position—there is little the state can do. The same is true if the medical director does insist and loses his job. When asked by a member of the Maryland investigating panel what he would do if a principal physician were fired by a home for attempting to carry out his duties, one licensing official was at first unable to answer. Then he replied, "I'd see that the home contracted with another physician." This is precisely the weakness of the position of medical director, which unfortunately has no more provision for stronger exercise of medical responsibility over the operations of a nursing home than the "principal physician" system.

In the inexcusable but continued absence of a way to guarantee physician supervision of and responsibility for the medical operations of nursing homes, medical review systems are urgently needed.

> In its simplest form, peer review consists of the periodic review of a number of a physician's cases by other physicians. The desired effect of peer review, sometimes called medical auditing, is to point out errors in judgment and mistakes in treatment and diagnosis so that such errors do not recur. . . . Studies of the effects of medical auditing reveal not only the beneficial effects of peer review, but also the great need for peer review in all phases of medical practice.[14]

A medical review team composed of respected physicians could be a strong force for insuring high levels of medical care on a statewide basis. When he realizes that his work is going to be evaluated by other doctors, a physician not only is able to learn from their knowledge, but also tends to administer care more conscientiously— just as motorists drive more carefully when a police car is cruising in the next lane. Such a review team would not be directly subject to influences of local physicians and nursing home operators, and, composed of prominent doctors, it could wield significant influence. The Moss amendments to the Medicare program, which Congress passed in 1967, directed the Social Security Administration to draw up regulations that would establish peer review in nursing homes. The SSA did not publish the regulations until April, 1970; during the three-year delay the SSA did nothing to encourage nursing homes to develop medical auditing before the law made it mandatory.

The Gould incident served tragically to expose the serious lack of medical supervision in that home and conceivably in thousands of other nursing homes where doctors visit individuals but ignore the home itself. Lack of medical supervision is a problem that doctors themselves have shown little interest in solving. In the absence of initiative from the medical profession, the Federal government and state public health officials

will have to fill the gap with strong and workable requirements for medical supervision of nursing homes. It
should not be "customary practice" for serious symptoms of illness to be written off as "common" among
the aged, nor for outbreaks of poisoning in a nursing
home to be treated with cavalier disregard by those
responsible.

The deaths at the Gould Convalesarium were not a
freak. The only thing freakish about the incident was
that it had not happened before, at Gould or another
home. Fifteen per cent of the nursing homes certified
for Medicare under the dangerous "substantial compliance" loophole—and probably a greater percentage
of those not receiving Federal funds—do not meet
food standards. Dietary inadequacy is fourth among the
deficiencies commonly noted by inspectors.

According to one HEW official, nursing home food
services frequently fail to control special diets. Puréed
foods, for example, are given to all patients, regardless
of who needs them; special diets are not given to those
who do need them, either through negligence or by design. Nursing homes also frequently attempt to save
money at the expense of quality by purchasing too-old
dairy products, poultry, fruit, and damaged canned
goods. Portions are often too small and starches are
served instead of meats and vegetables. Nursing home
food services often prepare and serve food poorly—
prepared foods sit for hours without refrigeration;
kitchens are operated without regard for sanitation.
Sometimes the homes fail to feed patients who are not
able to feed themselves.[15]

In a case such as the poisoning at the Gould home,
the effects of these deficiencies are easy to trace; death,
especially epidemic death, is conspicuous. There are
other effects which are more subtle, but serious nonetheless. In our visits to nursing homes, we observed lunch
trays loaded with unappetizing and tasteless packaged
sandwiches, a general dislike among the staff of feeding
patients, and food served puréed to all patients. Some
patients who eat puréed food or baby food become mal-
nourished because these foods do not contain enough
nutritive content for the average adult. We observed

food that should have been hot served stone-cold. The effects of these nuisances and others like them are not easy to trace, but indications are that they are grave.

As nursing home professionals point out, food is important to anyone regardless of his age. A patient does not automatically lose his love for food, his appetite, or his old eating habits as he ages. Moving into a nursing home can be a severe mental shock; to add the additional and needless shock of bad food badly served may be damaging to the patient.* The *Journal of Home Economics* notes that "the nutritional state is a mobile, fluid condition and may be modified adversely by many conditions and experiences of living. Stresses include changes in environment, social status . . . with the nutritional reaction being a refusal to eat, or else the other extreme of overeating." [16]

The symptoms of a deficient diet were described by John B. Martin, Commissioner for the Aging, before a Senate hearing in 1969: "Loss of appetite, fatigue, anxiety, irritability, loss of recent memory, insomnia, mild delusion states." Lack of vitamin B, he said, "produces severe depression and mental confusion, while protein deficiency is critical in transmitting nerve impulses." [17]

These symptoms are difficult to measure and often may not be traced to inadequate food. Strict enforcement of regulations and training of dietary staff and aides are minimal safeguards for nursing home patients. Only rarely, as in the wake of the epidemic at the Gould Convalesarium, is the public alerted to inadequacies in nursing home food services, but the problem remains severe and the consequences are often horrifying.

> My son was an invalid and died at the age of 21 after having spent five years in nursing homes. He was blind, immobile, and could not stand or feed himself. My husband is a mental patient. . . . In spite of the hardship, as I have another son to care for, I drove every day to

---

* We talked to one nursing home patient, a former dietician, who said that the reason nursing home food is poor is that it is too ambitious. "Instead of cooking good, easy, wholesome food," she said, "they try to dish out cocquille St. Jacques and other complicated things, and they ruin them."

see and care for my son, as the care was so poor in all
the nursing homes he was in. . . .

His death certificate speaks for itself. He contracted a
flu virus last fall and because he had received no care and
improper feeding, he died.

Four months before he died, I received a letter from
the * * * nursing home saying he was to be removed
immediately. When I asked why, I was told I broke all
the rules by feeding him between meals. . . . I never
fed him after that because I was afraid. The death certificate tells the rest. . . .

The death record from the State of Illinois listed as
"immediate cause" of death "pneumonia, terminal."
Under "other significant conditions contributing to death
but not related to cause given in Part I," the certificate
said, "malnutrition, severe, due to inadequate food intake."

THE ADMINISTRATOR

THE ESKIMOS USED TO FREEZE THEIR OLD
PEOPLE TO DEATH; WE BURY OURS ALIVE

Maybe the Eskimos were more merciful than we are. Ask
the old people in nursing homes across the country. A fast
death is a blessing we deny them. Yet we deny them a
human life, too. For these people life is an endless suc-
cession of deprivations. The food is poor and there's not
enough of it. A typical dinner at one Medicare approved
home consisted of one chicken wing and a scoop of
dried-up mashed potatoes. Insanitary conditions, lack of
medical care, uncaring, sometimes deliberately cruel attendants, lack of even the barest safety precautions against
fire or accident, are all facts of life for these patients.
Perhaps worst of all, there is nothing to do—day in and
day out—but wait for death to come.[1]

It is difficult and misleading to lump all nursing homes
together for discussion, just as it is unfair and incorrect
to speak of all older people as a single, all inclusive
group. Within just one type of nursing home—the Extended Care Facility—homes vary greatly in quality,
size, efficiency, atmosphere, organization of staff, and
administrators. Each home is a unique situation in itself,
linked with others mainly because it is reimbursed by the

Federal government for providing twenty-four-hour nursing services to eligible patients.

It is the administrator who determines the direction which a nursing home is to take. If he, or more often she, is a person with a good working knowledge of the problems and needs of older people, aware of the problems of the staff, sensitive to the fact that his home could very well be the last "home" for certain old people, and if he respects and appreciates older people, viewing them with the conviction that there is always possibility for improvement and recuperation, then every facet of his home will reflect this positive attitude. The reverse is also true. A negative attitude on the part of the administrator will be reflected by the staff and the quality of service.

There is no excuse for callous, brutal, or negligent treatment by the staff, if the administrator is attuned to the patient-staff relationship, and sets up each staff member's duty so that it does not exceed the person's limitations. There is no excuse for improper, insufficient diets if the administrator has enough experience in the health field to know how to utilize the services of a dietician properly. The administrator must have a basic knowledge of proper health care; he must also recognize his limitations in the field and be willing to seek sound professional advice when necessary. He must have a sound business knowledge and also be able to respond to and understand people in a field profoundly concerned with human beings. Patients are acutely sensitive to the attitudes of the administrator. He is the key person in the nursing home.

The crucial role of the administrator is obvious to anyone who has ever lived or worked in a nursing home. But for years, state and Federal regulations have almost totally neglected this central figure who, more than anyone else, determines the quality of the facility. In 1964, the Long-Term Care Subcommittee of the Senate Special Committee on Aging was given the responsibility of identifying major problem areas in the nursing home field. The Subcommittee was the first group to identify the administrator as the focal point in the efforts to improve standards in the nursing home, but not until 1967 were significant steps taken to insure the qualifications of the administrator, with passage of a federal law requiring licensing of nursing home administrators. The intent of Congress was to upgrade the educational qualifications of those administrators; however, a vigorous effort by the industry itself to control the licensing apparatus, combined with acquiescence by the Federal bureaucracy, meant that only a few mincing steps were taken toward stricter educational requirements.

The states had almost totally neglected the administrator in their regulations for licensing nursing homes. The regulations of thirteen states in 1967 did not even mention the administrator, and those of ten others did nothing more than refer to him by title. Twenty-eight states required no educational training or experience for the person holding this critical position. Only fourteen states required the administrator to be over twenty-one years of age; only twenty-two specified that he be in good physical health; and only nineteen made the point that he be in good mental health. Only nine required the administrator to be at least a high school graduate or the quivalent. Only twenty-one mentioned that he be of good moral character, and only nine indicated that he should have an interest in the welfare of the patients.[2] The failure of the states to demand qualified administrators was only too well reflected in what the nursing home industry supplied as the chief caretakers of the aged.

Samuel Levy, Director of the Massachusetts state nursing home licensing program, compiled statistics showing that among nursing home administrators in that state, "only 18 percent had completed college, 29 percent were high school dropouts; 1 percent had no formal education at all; and of these administrators, 85 percent supervised all personnel and 56 percent supervised nursing care directly."[3]

Conceivably, then, an eighteen-year-old high school dropout with a history of mental instability could be running a home for the elderly, with sole responsibility for hiring and directing personnel, managing food services, coordinating patient care activities, as well as handling business and financial arrangement and community relations.

The Federal government did little better than the states in setting standards for administrators. Initially, Medicare had only two specific requirements: that the administrator be twenty-one years old and work full-time at his job. The complete standards, which are so vague that they can be interpreted in any way, read as follows:

Sec. 405.1121(b)

(b) Standards; Full-time administrator—The governing body appoints a full-time administrator who is qualified by training and experience and delegates to him the internal operation of the facility in accordance with established policies. The factors explaining the standard are as follows:

(1) The administrator is at least 21 years old, capable of making mature judgments, and has no physical or mental disabilities or personality disturbances which interfere with carrying out his responsibilities.

(2) It is desirable for the administrator to have a minimum of a high school education, to have completed courses in administration or management and to have had at least 1 year of work experience including some administrative experience in an extended care facility or related health program.

In 1967, concern over the continuing poor quality of nursing home care, and the failure of the states to insure high standards, led to Congressional attempts to provide Federal leadership in upgrading these institutions. Chairman Moss of the Senate Long-Term Care Subcommittee, and Senator Edward Kennedy, the junior member of the Subcommittee, went to work on the problems. Senator Moss concluded that the states had not pushed for enforcement of sufficiently high standards as a condition of eligibility for Federal funds. His bill was designed to have the states impose certain minimum standards for homes wishing to receive Federal aid through Title XIX programs. Senator Kennedy focused his attention on the importance of the administrator in maintaining high standards in the nursing homes; his bill provided that the home have a licensed administrator before it could qualify for Federal financial assistance. Kennedy was particularly concerned with the lack of formal education of a large percentage of administrators, as revealed in Levy's study of Massachusetts administrators. His proposal, introduced in both May of 1966 and May of 1967, provided for licensing of nursing home administrators in each state by a board "representative" of the public, the professions, and the institutions concerned with long-term care.[4]

After undergoing certain alterations, the Kennedy bill became Section 1908 of the Social Security Act along with the Social Security Amendments of 1967. Changes in the redrafted bill provided for the creation of the National Advisory Council on Nursing Home Administration (NAC-NHA), which was to advise the Secretary on licensing standards. The Council had until July 1, 1969, for its first report to the Secretary and was to terminate December 31, 1971. Its composition, as prescribed in the subsection, was to include nine persons who were not employees of the U.S. government. They were to be appointed by the Secretary and to include "representatives of State health officers, State welfare directors, nursing home administrators, and university professors in public health or medical care administration.[5] The only guidelines in the amendment were that the administrator was to meet requirements of character, suitability, and either training or experience in the field of institutional administration. It was up to the NAC-NHA to recommend to the Secretary how the law was to be implemented.

Opposition of the nursing home industry to this amendment was obvious from the first. In fact, some people in HEW and elsewhere believe that the NAC-NHA was created as a compromise answer to the American Nursing Home Association's lobbying efforts to establish an advisory council of its own members to implement the licensing law—when they failed to succeed in killing the bill itself. The ANHA position was that any licensing program should cover all health care administration; if only nursing home administrators were to be licensed, the licensing board should be a peer group, as in the case of physician licensing boards. ANHA further stated that criteria and procedures for licensing should be developed prior to the establishment of state boards.[6]

The major fight over implementation of the law was about the composition of the group that would do the state licensing. Section 1908 says that if a state has a "healing arts licensing act," then the agency that administers that act must also license nursing home administrators. If there is no such designated agency, the licensing agency must be a board "representative of the professions and institution concerned with the care of chronically ill and infirm aged patients." [7] Interpretation of the word "representative" caused most of the confusion. According to Frank Frantz, a former member of the staff of the Senate Long-Term Care Subcommittee, the original intention of the Kennedy proposal was "to place the licensing function in a body which would be composed of nursing home administrators and other health professionals concerned with long-term care and which would be dominated by no one group." [8] The nursing home industry began to battle for a policy that would allow domination by the industry on the licensing boards.

The industry had cause to be concerned, since whatever form a state licensing board took, it could have a major impact on nursing homes. The function of the board was "the development and enforcement of standards, the issuance of licenses subject to revocation for cause, the investigation of complaints against administrators, and the gradual improvement of standards based on continuing study and investigation." [9] These powers were discomfiting: they might force nursing homes to spend money in ways which, though they might be good for the patients, would be bad for profits.

From the first, however, the National Advisory Council showed marked reluctance to encroach on what it considered the states' rights to administer Title XIX. It chose, therefore, not to recommend regulations but instead to develop a model law for the states to emulate if they wished. It was a course that was to prove costly for Federal influence in the licensing program. Neither the Council nor HEW considered the far more potent plan of guiding state action through the issuance of departmental regulations.

As a direct result of the Council's abdication of its powers to issue Federal regulations, the American Nursing Home Association was able to put itself in the enviable position of being the only major interest group that brought pressure to bear on the state legislatures, which were to pass the laws to administer Title XIX. The only other groups that might have had an interest in insuring high standards for administrators, the various state health agencies, had already lost interest, partly because the law did not relate administrator licensing to facility licensing. (The drafters of the bill had felt that the state agencies responsible for licensing facilities had shown such little enthusiasm for raising standards that they decided to vest administrator licensing in a different body.[10]) This meant that state health agencies, who had no responsibility for the program, took little interest in it. The major consequence of the division of licensing responsibilities was that ANHA was left alone on the field, the only powerful group with a reason to work to influence the state laws.

To blunt the effect of the National Advisory Council's model law, the American Nursing Home Association and the American College of Nursing Home Administrators (ACNHA) simply developed their own model laws. On several points, these laws were contrary to the provisions recommended by the Council. With their strong state and local lobby groups, the ANHA and the ACNHA were in a far better position to push for their recommendations.

The major conflict between the Council's model law and those recommended by the ANHA and its allies was interpretation of a "representative" board. The Council determined that "representative" meant the board should not have a majority from any one group. Its model law called for nine members, including four nursing home administrators, four health professionals from "other professions and institutions concerned with the care of the chronically ill and infirm aged," and one representative of "the public at large." The power of appointment was vested in the state governor, with the qualification that he consult the "appropriate" association or society before filling any vacancy.[11] In addition, the NAC-NHA model law provided for an advisory council to the licensing board composed of six administrators and "three others," as a compromise to the advocates of peer group review.[12]

The ANHA, on the other hand, drew up a model law that provided for a majority of nursing home administrators on the licensing board to insure the concept of peer group review. Neither the ANHA model law nor that recommended by the American College of Nursing Home Administrators provided any assurance that the board would be "representative" within the meaning of Section 1908.[13]

One of the primary aims of Section 1908 was the upgrading of educational qualifications of administrators. Accordingly, the NAC-NHA drew up the following provisions for the educational requirements: successful completion of high school, successful completion of at least a special course in nursing home administration, and a passing score on the examination given by the state licensing board. Candidates after 1971 would be required to have successfully completed two years of college level study; thereafter, the formal educational requirements would become possession of a B.A. degree in 1980 and possession of a master's degree in 1985.[14]

The Council made allowance for experience by providing that four years of work in nursing home administration could equal one year of posthigh-school education. The ANHA was strongly in favor of experience over formal education; the Council's equivalency formula was an attempt to mollify the Association.

The strong educational requirements in the Council's model law ultimately became its weakness so far as its ability to garner support from the nursing home industry. Opposition to these requirements, which appeared too stringent in the eyes of the industry, merely increased the energy with which the ANHA went about its drive to control the new licensing boards for administrators. The ANHA knew that the best way to control the standards for licensing was first to control the boards. It succeeded admirably, but not without the help of the Federal government.

The first step in turning over the administrator licensing procedure to the industry was the Council's recommendation not to issue regulations but simply to offer a suggested model law for the states' consideration. HEW agreed; thus, from the very beginning, the Federal government forfeited its best chance of carrying out the intention of Section 1908. It was a peculiar misjudgment, since the amendment was intended to be a response to the failure of the states to insure high standards for nursing homes. HEW was content to violate the intention of the law by simply turning the matter back to the states.

The second step in assuring the ineffectiveness of the new law was taken by the HEW Medical Services Administration, which develops and enforces Federal policies for all programs under medical assistance.[15] At this crucial time, MSA was inactive; it did not make a clear policy statement on nursing home licensing.[16] Nor does MSA apparently plan to do so, although Section 1102 of the Social Security Act specifically gives the agency the power to issue policy regulations. That the NAC-NHA failed to recommend mandatory regulations did not absolve MSA from its duty to guide the states, through substantive regulations, in implementing the new program. Even more than the failure of NAC-NHA, the silence of MSA opened the way for the states to implement the licensing program in any way they saw fit—or in any way that the powerful state chapters of the American Nursing Home Association dictated.

The Federal government's complicity did not end with these two serious acts of omission. Through the action of a top bureaucrat, HEW gave its unofficial stamp of approval to the nursing home industry control of the licensing boards.

The problem again lay with the definition of the key term "representative," which HEW did nothing to define through regulations, despite the law's intent and the recommendations of NAC-NHA that "representative" excluded a majority from the industry. Walter Kyle, past president of the Iowa Nursing Home Association, wrote to Mary Switzer, then head of HEW Social and Rehabilitation Services, to ask whether HEW would allow the nursing home industry to have a majority on the board. She wired Mr. Kyle on January 29, 1970, that HEW "would not object to a state board consisting of a simple majority of members representing one group, provided the remainder of the board membership is representative of the other professions and institutions concerned with the care of nursing home patients." [17]

Theodore Schuchat reprinted a copy of Miss Switzer's telegram in his column for the North American Newspaper Alliance for August 8–9, 1970:

Mr. Proctor N. Carter, Director
Division of Welfare
Department of Public Health and Welfare
State Office Building
Jefferson City Missouri 65101

Based on request David Walker Missouri Nursing Home Association to Mr. Thomas Laughlin Deputy Commissioner Medical Services Administration the content of the letter signed by Miss Mary Switzer Administrator Social and Rehabilitation Service date January 29, 1970, addressed to Mr. Walter Kyle 1020 Leavitt Street Waterloo Iowa is quoted below:

This is in response to our discussion yesterday concerning the membership of state boards to license nursing home administrators. Section 1908 (B) of the Social Security Act states that in the absence of a state agency responsible for licensing under the Healing Arts Licensing Act of the state, there must be "a board representative of the professions and institutions concerned with care of chronically ill and infirm aged patients" established to conduct the state nursing home administrator licensure program. In general, we believe that in establishing standards for an emerging profession, such as nursing home administrators, it is most desirable to have as broad a representation as possible in the composition of the board membership.

An overwhelming majority of representatives from any one professional or institutional group might tend to submerge the board with many preconceived concepts, some of which may already be outmoded by research and the rapid advances in the various disciplines represented in the fields of geriatrics and gerontology. The Department of Health, Education, and Welfare, however, would not object to a state board consisting of a simple majority of members representative of one group, provided the remainder of the board membership is representative of the other professions and institutions concerned with the care of nursing home patients. As an example, a nine-man board might consist of five nursing home administrators, with the remaining four members representative of such other professions as the medical, nursing, hospital administration, or educators in the health disciplines.

We trust that this will clarify the situation to your satisfaction. An identical telegram is being sent to Senator William Cason.[18]

The telegram indeed clarified the situation to the satisfaction of the nursing home industry, which immediately spread the word to other states. Nursing home lobbyists at once pushed through laws giving them control of the licensing boards in at least eleven states.[19] In Maryland, Governor Marvin Mandel appointed four owners of commercial nursing homes to his nine-man board, plus a salesman of ambulance service and nursing home supplies.[20] Also in Maryland occurred the omission, allegedly through a printing error, of a key paragraph from the regulations governing licensing. The deleted paragraph said: "Under no condition shall a majority of the board be composed of those having financial interests, other than as an employee, in one or more nursing homes whether designated as proprietary or nonprofit." [21]

In Oklahoma, all members of the regulatory board must be nominated by the Oklahoma Nursing Home Association, which reportedly occupies rent-free offices in the Capitol building.[22]

The outcome was predictable. According to NAC-NHA statistics on September 28, 1970, twenty-one of the thirty-four Medicaid jurisdictions with new licensing boards had a majority of members from the nursing home industry. Thirteen states went along with the recommendation by NAC-NHA that the board have a minority from the industry; two had not reported the composition of their boards; seven states authorized agencies to do the licensing and therefore had no boards;

four had a system whereby boards and agencies shared the licensing function.[23]

Contending forces in Massachusetts are still fighting over the licensing procedure to be adopted, and that state has not yet complied with the law.

The regulations for licensing that the states have adopted also indicate that the industry has succeeded in wielding strong influence, particularly with regard to the main purpose for which the law was passed: the upgrading of educational qualifications of administrators. No state has adopted the full recommendations made by the NAC-NHA in its model law. Four states require that by 1980 administrators will be required to have a college degree; five require that by 1975 administrators must complete two years of college; thirteen require that an administrator must complete high school.[24]

One state has adopted the Council's recommendation that four years of experience count as one year of post-high-school education. Two states say that two years of experience may count as one year of college; one state says that one year of experience may count as one year of college.[25]

The remaining states have not yet adopted laws under which to administer the law, as of this writing. But the pattern is clear. An attempt to upgrade the quality of care in nursing homes by requiring that administrators be educated or experienced in their profession fell flat, and neither the Federal government nor a majority of the states has more than minimal requirements for this vital position.

THE OWNERS

Federal law now requires that nursing home administrators be licensed, but not their owners. Yet owners of nursing homes, through entrance contracts and their final voice in decision-making, may be at least as important to their elderly patients as administrators, though less accessible. Owners are also farther removed from the public eye; in some cases, state licensing inspectors report that they cannot determine who the owner is. In the early days of nursing homes, the administrator and the owner were often the same person. Today the majority of owners are corporations or individuals who own a number of homes and are removed from immediate pressures from the community or government inspectors. One of the major problems of nursing homes today is holding owners accountable for the homes they operate.

The two major trends in nursing home ownership are large chain operations that have emerged in response to Medicare and other government programs that pour huge sums into nursing homes; and "hidden" chains, several nursing homes in different locations owned by the same individual or group. The older type of "ma and pa" nursing homes are dwindling; they constitute the major portion of homes that have withdrawn from participation in Medicare because they have not been able to make the necessary improvements.

Although state and Federal governments paid more than two-thirds of the two and a half billion dollars that went into all nursing homes in 1969, 90 per cent of all nursing homes are privately owned, profit-making operations. The only Federal regulation of ownership is a requirement that owners of 10 per cent or more of the interest in a nursing home report their ownership. The law is administered by the states under Federal reguluations. There are indications that stricter regulations are needed to prevent abuse by owners, particularly in the matter of entrance contracts that require patients to sign their possessions over to the nursing home for life—in effect making the patient a prisoner in the home.

Most of the homes with entrance contracts are sectarian. In some homes this practice was originally based on the convent tradition whereby a novice brought all her possessions to be used to support the residents of the convent. The patient entering such a nursing home may be required to sign a contract handing over all his possessions, including insurance policies, property, or any other investments.

Many contracts do not include provision for reversion of property after care has ended. Mr. and Mrs. K.

of Philadelphia had to threaten a lawsuit to get back
the property of Mrs. K.'s mother after she had signed
an "irrevocable" contract with a private nursing home
with a former association with the Presbyterian Church.

On entering the home, the patient signed a contract
turning over all her assets, plus a life insurance policy
for her burial and a deed to her burial plot, in return
for care for life.

> In view of the fact that the Home agrees to support the
> members of the Family for life, it is only right, and it is
> required, that those entering the Home execute, acknowl-
> edge, and deliver an assignment of all their assets to the
> Home, including insurances, investments, and etc., and
> also agree in writing, to assign and transfer, grant and
> convey, and pay over to the Home any and all property
> and rights in property which they may acquire, become
> vested with, or be entitled to after their admission.[1]

After three months, she became ill. She was in the infirmary for nearly two weeks before the home's doctor
sent her for X-rays to a hospital where it was found that
the patient had a bleeding ulcer and cancer. Concerned
for the type of medical care at the home, Mr. and Mrs.
K. took the patient to live with them and attempted to
get her property back. They were told by the home's
lawyer that she had signed everything over "irrevocably."
The home also demanded half of the former resident's
monthly Social Security checks, even though she was no
longer a patient.

It was only when the family threatened to sue the home
for negligence and the doctor for malpractice that the
home released the woman from the contract and returned her property, minus costs of care for three
months. Before the home did so, the former patient was
required to sign a document promising not to "pressure"
the home in any way.

Other patients do not fare so well. Bound by these
contracts, they cannot leave the institution without for-
feiting their property. Given the conditions of most
homes, and the difficulties of adjustment even in the
best facilities, the "irrevocable" entrance contract im-
poses a cruel restriction on the unhappy patient. If he
is dissatisfied, it also stifles his ability to demand better

care by threatening to leave the home. It grants the nursing home unreasonable control over the patient who, if he dares to leave, will be penniless.

The helplessness and dependency of the patients make it easy for nursing home owners to take advantage of them. Legal means to allow an entrance contract to be broken by both the home and the patient should be considered by Congress and state legislatures. In making a case for including owners under the Federal licensing law, Theodore Schuchat reports:

> The new law's [licensing of administrators] loopholes are exemplified by the case of Sossin System, Inc., a retirement hotel-nursing home drugstore chain headquartered in Miami Beach, Fla. This fast-growing firm is headed by one Michael Sossin, who discusses his companies with the candor and clarity of a used-car salesman, which is what he was before getting into the more profitable nursing home business.
>
> Advertisements for the Blackstone Retirement Residence, adjoining one of his nursing home and drugstores, call him "Dr. Michael Sossin, Executive Director."
>
> He is similarly styled by the signs outside this place of business on his office door and atop his imposing desk, as well as on the many commendatory placques and scrolls that adorn his walls. One is a certificate of membership in the Gerontological Society, a reputable professional group.
>
> His doctorate degree is in law, however, not medicine or gerontology. It was granted more than a decade ago by Cookman-Bethune College, a Daytona Beach, Fla., institution that lacks a law school and confers no earned doctorates. There is no record of Sossin's attendance at this or any other seat of higher learning.
>
> Sossin is an active member of many civic, religious and fraternal groups, though not of the Better Business Bureau of Southern Florida. He operated the Blackstone Retirement Residence, a pink stucco relic of the 1920's, under the aegis of the Sossin's Foundation for Geriatric Research until his lawyer advised him to create a taxable corporation.
>
> Sossin is not unacquainted with the courts in his community. On February 28, 1963, he and his corporation filed papers to cancel a $1.7 million mortgage on the Blackstone Hotel. Their suit asserted that the actual purchase price was $475,000, the higher amount having been

stated in 1957 only to avoid taxes and a law against usurious loans.

More pertinent to his business of caring for older people, however, was Case No. 39759-B before Dade County Judge Frank Dowling in August 1956. As guardian of the assets of the late Mamye L. Wolf, Sossin pawned her diamond jewelry, then reclaimed the gems from the pawnshop without informing the courts. Upon confessing perjury, he was replaced as guardian of this oldster's assets but suffered no other penalty.

Spokesmen for local social service agencies and senior citizens' organizations say that Sossin ingratiates himself with many of his residents and patients, some of whom are then moved to name him as executor or beneficiary of their modest estates.

In one case of this kind, when Isaac Cohen died on November 25, 1958, in one of Sossin's establishments, his death certificate was signed by his landlord, as a "lawyer." With evidence in hand of Cohen's demise, Sossin at once took charge of the decedent's $8,800 account at the Miami Beach Federal Savings and Loan Association.

Cohen made Sossin the cosigner of his "working trust" account of which Cohen had full control until his death, without awaiting settlement of his estate or other legal formalities.[2]

In his article Schuchat goes on to point out that there is no protection for the public from Sossin and others like him.

At present, neither Federal nor State laws restrain Sossin and his ilk. The new Federal law requires that nursing home licensees be "of good character . . . and otherwise suitable," but owners are not licensed, only their hired managers.

No law prevents nursing home operators from handling funds of their patients, serving as executives of their estates or receiving bequests under their wills. Yet these businessmen are uniquely placed to flimflam or coerce their lonely, dependent "guest," many of whom are senile or easily confused.

Clearly, the new nursing home licensure law is only the first little legislative step towards decency and morality in this dark corner of the American marketplace.[3]

A major new trend in nursing home ownership has been the entrance of corporations with large chain op-

erations, which have largely accounted for the unprece-
dented building boom in response to Medicare. Between
1967 and 1969, the number of nursing homes in this
country increased from thirteen thousand to over twenty-
three thousand. The new Federal programs, with guaranteed reimbursements, opened up a rich field for the
profit-oriented corporations seeking greener pastures for
diversification.

In a series on the rapidly expanding public ownership
in the nursing home field, *Barron's* reported in 1969
that nursing homes

> stand for the hottest investment around today. . . . Com-
> panies never before near a hospital zone—from builders
> like ITT's Sheraton Corporation, National Environment
> and Ramada Inns, to Sayre & Fisher, Irvington Place and
> Computer Research—have been banging on the industry's
> door. More significantly for investors, nursing home oper-
> ators have been selling shares to the public at a dizzying
> rate. . . .[4]

On February 10, 1969, *Barron's* reported that "at
least 50 such equities were on the market or in registra-
tion; new filings currently average one or two a week.
The 50 can lay claim to nearly 800 homes for the aged
and infirm (including units on the drawing board), with
total patient capacities approaching 100,000 beds."[5] By
the time the last article in the series appeared on March
17, *Barron's* had to update its chart to include twenty-
four more corporations on the market.[6]

In the 1970's, this boom has leveled off as corporations have become concerned with government regulations involving expenditures which make nursing
homes less of a major money-making enterprise than
they first appeared. This building boom had its good
side, because the United States *does* need more nursing
homes. On the whole, however, it has bred more evil
than good: growth has brought chaos without improvement, and has aggravated our already critical shortage
of qualified personnel to staff nursing homes. A spank-
ing new facility staffed by surly aides and minimally
competent nurses is not much good.

Even at the beginning, companies that simply plunged
into the nursing home business without knowledge or

experience in the health field ran into problems of administration. *Barron's* reporter J. Richard Elliott, Jr., found that "of the host of factors affecting the profitable development and operation of nursing homes . . . probably the key component is management inexperience." [7] He reports that

> demand for experienced administrators far exceeds the supply; to make matters worse for the nursing homes, general hospitals usually attract the cream. In consequence, nursing home companies, from the smallest to the biggest . . . must hire and train recruits wherever they can be found.[8]

One chain, American Institutional Developers, told *Barron's* that it put every new administrator through a one-year course of instruction.

> Then we equip him with our nurse's procedure manual, our book on dietary proprietary procedures and a number of other policy guides and send him out to the facility three months before it's ready to open. He gets to know his business backwards and forwards by the time the first patient arrives.[9]

The company did not explain how one can get experience in medical care without patients to care for.

Elliott reports that many operations have courses for new administrators lasting from three to six months. But he also reveals that top management, which provides the training for the administrators, are no better versed in the problems of running nursing homes than are the newly recruited administrators. He quotes one top company official of Medicenters, whose two major stockholders and officers are chairman and vice-chairman of the board of the Holiday Inn Corporation,* as saying, "You learn this business from your mistakes, and the top management has to learn it the same way." [10] Another company official was more direct: "You might say it was the blind leading the blind around here for a while." [11]

---

* Kemmons Wilson, chairman of the board of Holiday Inn, is vice-chairman of the board of Medicenters. Wallace Johnson, vice-chairman of Holiday Inn, is chairman of Medicenters. There is no corporate connection.

The reporter found that new chain operations headed
by managers with even the slightest experience in the
health field are the rare exceptions. For example,
Extendicare, one of the industry's three biggest concerns,
is managed by a "co-founding quartet of crackerjack
young lawyers and accountants, not one of whom had
been near a nursing home or hospital (except as a
patient) until two or three years ago." [12] Elliott concluded, "Clearly, top management in the nursing home
business, taken as a whole, is a motley group. The same
is true at the day-to-day, unit-by-unit, working level.
Second-echelon expertise . . . apparently is a commod-
ity almost as scarce as the Rh-negative factor." [13]

Industry leaders find nursing home administrators in
strange places, according to *Barron's*. " 'One of our
ablest administrators,' Four Seasons President Jack
Clark likes to say, 'is a former bakery foreman.' And at
Medicenters in Memphis, a spokesman recalls that 'the
best one I've run into used to operate a filling station.' " [14]

The *Barron's* reporter is skeptical of these industry
claims: "Nevertheless, some of the evidence to date
leaves room for doubt. From pumping gas or selling
auto parts to administering a 100-bed extended care
facility—or managing a string of dozens of them—
seems, at least to some observers, a long stretch
indeed." [15]

Desire for profits may lead owners to seek administrators who are good businessmen; the same desire may
prove a negative influence on the patient's demand for
trained personnel and other costly services. Additional
pressures on the owner are needed to insure that patient
care does not give way to profit-making. As nursing
home ownership shifts more and more to the invisible
or distant owner, it is increasingly difficult for the public
or patients to hold owners accountable. The requirement to register owners of 10 per cent or more of the
stock in a home has not worked to make all owners
visible. Val Halamanderis, chief counsel to the Senate
Committee on Aging, points out that owners may transfer stock to their wives or children in order to conceal
their ownership. For example, a married man with four
children could effectively control 54 per cent of the stock

in a nursing home without having to tell anyone. But when abuses occur, or when nursing homes are negligent, the public must be able to hold owners legally responsible.

Such practices as irrevocable entrance contracts, inexperienced and often unknown ownership, and haphazard growth without regard for the medical consequences—these are inconsistent with the public interest, with the proper operation of a health care facility, with the use of Federal funds for what amounts to a subsidy of an already very profitable industry, with common decency.

THE PERSONNEL

THE AIDE

When I arrived at the home for my first shift, the head nurse told me that I was to work on the intensive care floor. I reminded her that I had had absolutely no experience whatsoever in nursing, but she just said, "You'll learn." [1]

The job of aide is probably the most demanding and least rewarding of all positions in the nursing home. Certainly it is the least rewarding in monetary terms. Nursing aides have only recently been included under Federal minimum wage laws; as of February, 1971, their wages reached the national minimum of $1.60 an hour.

The low wage does not reflect the importance of the nursing aides, who have the most extensive and intimate contact with the patients of all nursing home personnel. Because of the critical shortage of nurses, and because Federal standards require that only one nurse be employed, aides take on major responsibilities for daily patient care and indeed become central figures in the patient's world. Their duties usually include helping the patient to the bathroom, washing and dressing him, changing the bed and cleaning the room, bringing the bedfast patient his meals and sometimes feeding him. There is also the chore of doing the laundry in some nursing homes and performing other housekeeping tasks.

Moreover, the aides must have the skill and knowledge necessary to recognize problems that require a nurse's attention.

Low wages and hard work account in part for the high turnover among aides. Department of Labor statistics estimate that the annual turnover rate for all nursing personnel in homes approaches 60 per cent. For aides and orderlies, the rate is 75 per cent; registered nurses, 71 per cent; licensed practical nurses, 35 per cent; and administrative and supervisory nursing personnel, 21 per cent.[2] Many aides work in homes only to build up references to get a better job, but the high turnover rate also reflects management practices. Aides who have left jobs in nursing homes generally point to its depressing atmosphere and inadequate patient care as often as to overwork and low wages. One twenty-one-year-old aide wrote:

> There are sixty patients where I work and they are nearly all old and suffering, not so much from the cares which afflict their bodies but from the monotony and loneliness which living in a convalescent home implies. I found this kind of suffering even penetrating the first nursing home I worked at, where the patients' physical care was more than adequate and where some attempt was made to involve them in social activities. . . . I soon came to realize though that the patient care at this particular rest home was the exception rather than the rule. As soon as one enters the sanitarium where I work now, one is hit by the sense of meaninglessness in the lives of the patients. . . . Many times I felt that I could stand it no longer and that working for such people was only perpetuating the conditions. But someone has to do it. . . .[3]

The duties of the aide may be largely menial, but there is skill involved in the handling of patients. Yet few homes have even minimal training for new aides, or minimal requirements for hiring; most homes seem glad to take what they can get. Jim Treloar, a reporter for the Detroit *News,* posed as a mentally unstable person with a criminal record when he applied for a job at a nursing home. He was hired immediately. Although our task force took jobs for which we had absolutely no experience, no member of this study was given any training other than the opportunity to watch a nurse or another aide at work. Medicare standards call for the "training and orientation" of all new personnel, but the "continuing inservice educational program" set down in the standards is farcical in reality. In addition, no records are kept by Federal agencies regarding training or practices in hiring aides. Our own observation, along with letters and accounts that have come to us during the study, indicate that few nursing homes have any program of instruction for aides.

This is true despite the difference that a competent or an incompetent aide can make in a patient's adjustment to the nursing home. The aide's intimate, daily contact with patients has a tremendous effect on the patients' mental and emotional health and, directly or indirectly, on their physical health as well. The need for teaching aides skills in handling patients is obvious.

Training and supervision of the attitudes toward patients is just as important as learning the skills of the job. Brutality on the part of the staff toward nursing home patients is reported so frequently that it cannot be entirely written off as the hallucinations of the aged. In our firsthand experience in nursing homes, we witnessed a shocking lack of sensitivity as well as a lack of competence, particularly among the aides.

The following are excerpts from letters written to Congressman David Pryor of Arkansas after his exposé of the nursing home situation in the Washington, D.C., area:

From Arkansas:

> Brutality is another thing that goes on. She has one aide that tells her how she beat the patient and let her get by with anything including murder because once she pushed a patient down and she broke her hip. . . .

From Texas:

> The first thing as anyone knows, the aides do most of the work and they make $1.45 an hour and have 15 patients to care for and God knows there cannot be justice done, therefore they don't get half the care they need.

From "a nurse from New York who cares":

> I have also found that many of the people that work

these jobs as aides are resentful of having to do it. Many of them have warped minds and the teasing and the threats that these old people have to endure is beyond belief. The fear in the eyes of the stroke victims when certain aides care for them is proof enough.

From Florida:

I have seen and reported aides [who] push and hit the aged, steal their food and money and clothes. I once saw an aide throw a fork at a crippled old lady because the aides did not want to set the table at which her friends were eating their lunch.

No address given:

There is a lot of cruelty here besides what I have been subjected to. They tie them in their chairs and beds and I saw one white attendant slap a 95-year-old lady in the face six times and another take her by the shoulders and shake her as hard as she could.

From Texas:

It was a prank for revenge for one shift to load the patients with laxatives so the next shift would have to work cleaning up. One of the patients was so weak she was almost dead from laxatives and fleet enemas.

From Rhode Island:

Before he died he told me they treated him like an animal such as "oh, shut up" and they shoved him around in bed.

From New Jersey:

Several times I found people lying on the floors and when I reported this to the nurses at the nursing station I was told that they would take care of that patient when they got around to it. I found that this was very common along with other things such as the nurses on the evening and night shifts turning off the call system so they do not have to be bothered since many of the nurses and aides sleep on the evening and night shifts.

From Pennsylvania:

I have seen them lay in bed till noon wet, begging for a bedpan. Sometimes if they caused any trouble, a needle took care of that.

From Texas:

[I saw] Ambulatory, incontinent patients walking around, soaking wet, tramping fecal matter and urine which the 2 nurses never seemed to get the time to clean up.

From California:

The patients were never kept clean. One day [as] I sat on the sun porch, one of the elderly picked up her own bowel movement and threw it away from her as best she could. When I went looking for help, I found at least 6 aides, closeted in a room chatting, while the patients relieved themselves on the sun porch, because they could no longer wait for help. And this was not an isolated incident.

From Indiana:

One lady had cried to go to the bathroom and they just said let her wait. Then if she is put on the stool, she almost passes out before they go get her off, you see, she can't walk.

From Colorado:

I needed help to turn over and also have a bedpan. If I turned on my light more than once or twice during the night the aide would take it away and say "let it go in the bed." She would rather clean the bed than to bring the bedpan. That doesn't make sense. Furthermore, I had no desire to lie in such a mess. Some of the aides would wipe out the bedpan with a washcloth which would have later been used on the face had I not stopped it.

From California:

I went by one afternoon after work to pick up my daughter just as the food trays were being delivered. One of the men aides said to one of the girl aides, "It's your night to feed old Annie," and the girl refused, and he said "Well, I ain't gonna feed her." With that the girl dumped her tray back on the cart and said, "Well, as far as I'm concerned all the bastards can go hungry."

From Connecticut:

I have witnessed these aides throwing patients' food down the toilet because the patient might be a slow eater. If the patient complained they didn't know what they were talking about because they were senile or any other excuse they could think of at the time.

From Massachusetts:

> The home I work in is beautiful on the surface. One visiting it is really impressed by surface appearances but one has to work or live in it to know what really goes on behind the scenes. This home is equipped with patient buzzers but the aides (especially 4 P.M.–12 P.M.) pay no attention to them. There should be at least one aide at the desk at all times to answer these calls for help and get the nurses' aides to go and do her job.

From Arkansas:

> I was under the assumption that only a nurse could dispense medicine. On one occasion a maid came into one of the rooms, with a handful of pills and capsules and asked one of the elderly women there if she knew which medicine was hers, resulting in a possible death if erroneous medicine were taken.

From Texas:

> I'm uneducated and allowed to fix medicine and even give [medication] through tubes.

Because no statistical data are available on nursing home aides, there is no way to know how many homes provide training or how many simply turn over their patients to inexperienced staff. The letters above are one indication that a problem exists. No study has been made to indicate how extensive the problem may be, but everyone contacted by members of this task force confirmed that poor care by nursing home aides is a serious problem.

Ther are ways to train and attract competent aides; manpower programs, "new careers" programs, and vocational education already exist. There is also a training requirement in Medicare standards. But as long as the standard is not enforced, and the programs are not used, elderly people will continue to suffer needless and intolerable abuses at the hands of untrained aides.

THE NURSE

In 1961, the American Nurses Association (ANA) established a group devoted to geriatric nursing in an effort to improve its quality.[4] For the ANA to give attention to a nurse's specific clinical role was a revolutionary step that indicates just how low the quality was. Traditionally, nurses who took care of the elderly were considered a step below other nurses. Their duties were not clearly defined; they might wash dishes or mop floors. They were not usually regarded as professionals with special skills but as caretakers with fewer skills than those required in other areas of nursing. In the 1950's there were still no books or pamphlets on geriatric nursing. Nurses for the elderly, and retired nurses who commonly took elderly people to live in their homes (the origin of the present-day nursing home), relied on experience and little else. The lack of definition and identification of the special training skills required for treating the aged meant that the elderly were generally shortchanged with less competent nurses.

By 1968, 15,570 registered nurses were members of the Geriatric Nursing Division of the ANA. Within two years, by September, 1970, the number had more than doubled—37,811. This progress is as admirable as it is astonishing, but even if we make the questionable assumption that all these nurses have excellent skills, elderly patients are still in serious trouble. While the shortage of registered nurses and licensed practical nurses is general throughout American medicine, the shortage of geriatric nurses is critical. If every member of the Geriatric Division worked in a nursing home, there would still be only one and a half nurses for each of the twenty-four thousand nursing homes in the country—with none left over for hospitals, clinics, doctors' offices, and home-care services. Twice as many nurses are needed just to supply each home with one geriatric nurse twenty-four hours a day—again, with none left over for medical services outside nursing homes.

The facts of the matter are that most of the nurses in nursing homes are not geriatric nurses, and that, to qualify for Federal assistance, a home needs only one full-time registered nurse, and one licensed practical nurse on the premises when the registered nurse is not there (conditions that are not always met—17 per cent of the nursing homes receiving Medicare funds do not attain these low heights), and that, as our experience taught us, the nurses in homes are not of the high quality that is needed. Moreover, the registered nurse in a home is so tied down by law and routine medical duties that he or she is often useless as far as other duties are concerned. Only a registered nurse is permitted to keep clinical records on patient care—an enormously time-consuming task—and only she is permitted to administer medicine. Although these laws are often flouted, the registered nurse still has too much to do; if the law were scrupulously obeyed—as it should be, for the safety of the patients—homes with only one registered nurse would never get the full benefit of her services. The problem is made more acute by the maldistribution of nurses. Good homes have several registered nurses, enough to care for their patients well; the rest may have only one R.N. for as many as one hundred patients.

The quality of nursing care naturally reflects the attitudes of the nursing home owners and administrators. Since registered nurses earn more money than practicals or aides, a nursing home operator with his eye glued to the profit chart is likely to employ as few as possible. Similarly, a good nurse whose services are much in demand will generally avoid such homes, where conditions are unpleasant and work is uninteresting, harried, and limited by the administration's obsessive cost-consciousness.

The nurses and the ANA are not the villains of this piece. Congress for establishing low standards, the Social Security Administration for failing to enforce them, and the nursing home owners who cling to the letter of an inadequate law and shun the logical proposition that a *nursing* home should provide good *nursing* care—these, and the ever-present, dangerous American distaste for old age, are the villains. The recognition that the needs of the elderly require special study is a step toward better health care for the aged. The fact that recognition by the nursing profession came as late as 1961—and then in conjunction with new national attention to the health problems of the elderly—indicates the need for more public impact on the medical professions in general. In their support for national health insurance proposals, nurses have shown more responsibility than physicians and nursing home operators; for this the aged and the nation can be grateful. The pity is that good nursing care is still a distant target.

THE DOCTOR

The role of the doctor in the nursing home is an ambiguous one. The Federal government initially recognized the need for close attendance by physicians in nursing homes that provide postoperative care by attempting to locate Extended Care Facilities in hospitals. But there were few hospitals with bed space for the ECF; nor has there been an impressive increase of the hospital-based ECF since the advent of Medicare.* What this has usually meant for the nursing home patient is removal from the direct care of a doctor. For some, it means a brief visit from the physician once or twice a month. For others, it means little direction or supervision of their care on a day-to-day basis, prescriptions that run too long or are not refilled, changes in conditions that are not met by changes in prescribed treatment. While the nursing home staff at times may be at fault for not reporting a patient's condition to the attending physician, evidence also points to the fact that doctors are not available as often or as consistently as the medical needs of the patients demand. This is indicated by the difficulty we observed in getting in touch with doctors in emergencies, the complaints of patients about the infrequent and hurried visits from their doctors, and statistics on "gang visits" by physicians to nursing homes.

In one nursing home we visited, a woman, partially paralyzed by a stroke, had sores on her upper leg caused by the rubbing of her catheter tube. Her ointment had not been refilled before it ran out and could only be refilled with a doctor's prescription. Although Miss X. was crying

* According to the Social Security Administration, there were some one hundred hospital-based Extended Care Facilities when Medicare was enacted. There are now over six hundred, out of more than forty-five hundred certified Extended Care Facilities.

with pain, the nurse said resignedly, "It's impossible to get hold of a doctor on a Friday night. We will have to wait until Monday." [5]

The General Accounting Office of the Federal government found that some doctors visit from seventy to ninety patients a day, in several different nursing homes. If eight full hours were spent with patients, this meant each patient got an average of six minutes with the doctor. Full visiting fees were charged for these "gang visits." A GAO audit of homes in the Cleveland, Ohio, area found that on one day,

> Medical Doctor A visited 71 patients, 68 in one nursing home while the other three visits were at separate locations close to the nursing home. Medical Doctor B billed and was paid for visits to 90 patients on February 10, 1966, and to 79 patients on February 27. For further analysis, we plotted the locations of the indicated visits for February 27, a Sunday, on a map of the Cleveland area. We found that 73 of the 79 indicated visits were in four nursing homes (30, 27, 14 and 2 visits made to the four homes, respectively) close to one another. The other six visits were at separate locations, two visits about five miles southeast of the nearest nursing home, two visits about seven miles west of the nursing home and one visit near the nursing home. We estimate the travel between these locations would involve a distance of about 30 miles within the Cleveland metropolitan area.[6]

The Senate Finance Committee's report of February, 1970, also referred to the practice of "gang visits," which the GAO audit report had apparently failed to halt. The Committee staff recommended that "to avoid, at least to some extent, costly and often medically unnecessary 'gang visiting,' amounts allowed should be reduced for multiple visits, on the same day to patients in the same facility." [7]

An employee of a nursing home wrote:

> One doctor would come in on Sunday once in a while with his two small children to see his patients' charts and then leave. I used to think that he was paying them an extra visit and I mentioned how nice it was that he found the time to inquire about his patients. The L.P.N. replied that the visits on Sunday were the only ones he ever made

and that all he did was look at the charts and leave. . . .[8]

A serious omission of the medical profession has been the failure to take the responsibility for the nursing home as a whole. Though doctors are occasionally critical of nursing homes, there is no sign that they have taken the initiative to upgrade them or provide adequate medical direction for the total nursing home program. That they believe their responsibility ends with individual patients in a nursing home was made all too clear by the tragic deaths of twenty-five patients at the Gould Convalesarium in Baltimore.*

A panel that investigated the case for the Maryland Health Department found that no doctor considered himself responsible for reporting the epidemic, as required by state law, nor for the general conditions that affected the health of all the patients. The doctors frankly admitted that there was no formal communication between them and the nursing home staff; they generally visited their own patients without consulting with the nurses. The "principal physician" at the Gould Convalesarium hastened to tell the investigating committee that his title did not mean that he was responsible for conditions in the nursing home in general.

A committee of the Maryland Medical Society found the attending physicians guilty of violating two state laws but no prosecutions were made. The reasons, explained Dr. Matthew Tayback of the Maryland Health Department, were that officially no single physician was responsible for the totality of health care at the home, there was nothing "malicious" found in the actions of the doctors, and there was nothing "contrary to usual medical practice."[9] The Maryland Health Department is now developing a new standard for its nursing homes that will require a "medical director" who will be clearly responsible for the totality of medical care in a nursing home. The public health official emphasized that at present there is no one with this responsibility. He added, "It is unfortunate that an incident of this type was required to bring the situation to our attention."[10]

---

* For a complete discussion, see Chapter 3.

The reason that physicians themselves have not recognized the need for taking responsibility is indicated in Tayback's comment that installing a medical director "is a sticky business because of the private doctors' feelings about having someone over them." In the Gould case, twenty-five patients paid with their lives for such professional jealousy.

The role of the doctor caring for the elderly needs more professional emphasis in the medical schools. Talking to students and to doctors who teach at medical schools, we found that geriatrics is among the least popular courses. The tendency seems to be for medical students to look to fields in which more striking advances may be made, or in which children are healed or widespread diseases dealt with. A young intern is likely to feel greater satisfaction saving a child's life than by prolonging the last few weeks or years of an old patient in a nursing home. Economic factors are also present. A young doctor building his reputation and his clientele is more likely to pick younger patients who will need his help over a long period of time, and who may bring their children to him in the future, than older nursing home patients. Because of these human and economic pressures on young doctors, the role of the medical school is vital in persuading more doctors to become concerned with the special problems of the aged.

DRUGS

The American Medical Association has issued at least six pamphlets to inform the public about drug addiction among the young. The "drug problem" to most people relates almost solely to the young. The obvious opportunities for abuse and misuse of drugs among the elderly, who consume more drugs than any other segment of the population, are largely ignored. One California physician, when told of an elderly woman's addiction to Percodan, replied, "She's an old lady. Let her enjoy it."

The large quantity of drugs consumed by elderly patients in nursing homes requires special measures of regulation; and there are requirements under Medicare conditions of participation for the proper administration and storage of drugs. But government statistics suggest widespread carelessness in the handling of drugs in nursing homes. Drugs are administered incorrectly or not at all, drugs prescribed by physicians are allowed to continue too long, or too many drugs are prescribed, or drugs are administered that have not been prescribed by a physician. Even more widespread is the practice of keeping patients under sedation to reduce the demands on nursing home staff. Numerous letters citing this abuse have been forwarded to members of our task force. Experts in the field also affirm that excessive sedation is a serious problem in nursing homes. When asked whether he had seen any new drug experiments, a medical student inspecting nursing homes in Washington, D.C., said, "No, but in the homes I've seen, almost any drug is experimental." [1]

A 1970 General Accounting Office audit, *Continuing Problems in Providing Nursing Home Care and Prescribed Drugs Under the Medicaid Program in California,* revealed the alarming extent of the failure to administer drugs correctly. A review of one month's medical records of 106 Medi-Cal patients at 14 nursing homes showed that: "311 doses were administered in quantities in excess of those prescribed; and 1,210 prescribed doses were not administered." [2] The nursing home administrators' explanation to the auditors was that "(1) there were errors on the patients' medical charts and the medications had been correctly administered and (2) the medications were given on an as-needed basis and, in some cases, the patients did not need the medications at the time it was supposed to have been administered." [3]

Interestingly, GAO auditors found the same abuses in 1966 when they looked at nursing home care provided to California welfare recipients. Auditors "made a random selection of 36 welfare patients, 3 in each of the 12 nursing homes visited, and compared the nurses' records of medications and treatment for about a 3-month period with the doctors' order for the patients." [4]

In 11 homes, we found that the records indicated that 51 medications involving 1,208 dosages were not administered at the frequency ordered by the doctors—76 more dosages were administered than the number ordered by the doctors for the time periods involved and 1,132 dosages ordered by the doctors were not recorded as having been administered to the patients.[5]

Having found that the same malpractices pointed out in 1966 were continuing in 1970, the GAO auditors were characteristically low-key in stating their disturbing conclusion: "Actions taken by HEW and the state to correct the previously reported problems were generally ineffective." [6]

It is not entirely facetious to suggest that if nursing home patients were allowed to administer their own drugs they would be more likely to get them correct. At the International Gerontological Association meeting in Washington, in 1969, a study was reported in which elderly patients showed a self-administration error rate markedly lower than the known nurse-administration rate. Twenty elderly patients "with the quite significant illnesses *listed*" self-administered "placebo" medication.

During one week they each made three self-administrations per day; that is, a white tablet twice a day and a blue-white capsule every morning. During a second week, four of these subjects made six self-administrations per day; that is, in addition to the twice a day tablet and once a day capsule, they also took a second white tablet, three times per day. The rating was done during the physician's visit by simply counting the medications remaining in the bottles.

The table shows that 14 errors were made during 588 self-administration opportunities. This error rate of 2.5% is quite small in comparison to the known nurse-administration error rate of 1 in 7 administrations; that is, 14%.[7]

But the fact is that it is the responsibility of the nursing home and of the physician to see that the patient gets the drug he needs, and does not get what he does not need. What happens all too often is that the patient is placed in a "holding pattern": he is kept docile by being given too many drugs for too long. In this way, both physicians and nursing homes subject patients to pharmaceutical overkill.

The quantity of drugs prescribed for nursing home patients is described as a problem by a nursing home inspector in Montgomery County, Maryland. Mrs. Virginia Maxwell said that some patients have written orders for up to fifteen drugs.[8] Her view is corroborated at the state level by Mrs. Virginia Westbrook, R.N., of the Missouri Department of Public Health and Welfare:

> I wish to emphasize that there has always been an unusually large number of medications ordered for the elderly patients in our nursing homes. I can see no difference in this since 1957. The one individual I spoke to you about is now deceased, but when he was being cared for there were 28 different drugs ordered. Another lady in another home had 11 ordered for her. *These are not unique situations, but samples.*[9] (Emphasis added.)

The duration of prescriptions can be equally alarming. "Drug prescriptions tend to run forever, or as long as the patient lasts. I've seen prescriptions six years old on some medical charts," says Associated Press writer Jim Polk, who did a five-part series on nursing homes in September, 1969.[10]

Both the quantity of drugs prescribed and their duration, traditionally the responsibility of the physician, should be checked by Medicare's Condition of Participation for Extended Care Facilities which states: "The charge nurse and the prescribing physician together review monthly each patient's medications." It continues: "Medications not specifically limited as to time or number of doses, when ordered, are automatically stopped in accordance with written policy approved by the physician or physicians responsible for advising the facility on its medical administrating policies." However, the reluctance of many physicians to visit nursing homes, and the "gang-visits" by those who do, make it unlikely that such reviews are made regularly or that automatic stop orders are watched closely by the prescribing physician.[11] According to a former nursing home administrator quoted by James Treloar in his article on nursing homes in the Detroit *News:*

> The doctors, they were supposed to prescribe these drugs. But they never did.
> They'd come in and here'd be all the doctors' daily reports. The doctors didn't make them out. The nurses did. The doctors just came in and signed these things.

They never read them. They didn't even look at the dead patients.[12]

Even the conscientious physician may overprescribe. Dr. Robert Butler, a gerontologist, cites the case of a seventy-four-year-old lady who was given Mellaril to calm her before a cataract operation. The dose was increased after the operation; she seemed to be increasingly senile and was given more and more drugs. When the doctor took her off all medication, she quickly returned to normal.

But it is nursing homes, not physicians, who have most to gain when patients are under sedation. Frank Frantz, Assistant to the Commissioner of the Medical Services Administration, suggests guidelines for choosing a nursing home: "Observe other patients. Are a number dressed in street clothes and actively occupied, walking around, chatting or reading? Too little patient activity may be a sign that sedatives and tranquilizers are being substituted for genuine care." [13]

The former nursing home administrator interviewed by Treloar expands on the general practice Frantz warns of:

> A layman doesn't know what to look for in a nursing home. He walks in and sees a patient is nice and quiet and he thinks this guy is happy. And the nurse tells him: "This is John. John is one of our best patients. He sits here and watches television."
>
> But you just take a look at John's pupils, and you'll see what condition John is in. John is so full of thorazine that it's coming out his ears. Thorazine—that's a tranquilizer they use. It's a brown pill. It looks like an M & M candy.
>
> The nursing home where I worked kept at least 90 percent of the patients on thorazine all the time. They do it for the money. If they can keep John a vegetable, then they don't have to bother with him. They never have to spend anything to rehabilitate him.[14]

The General Accounting Office audit of care received by California welfare recipients states: "The nurses' records showed that the third patient was receiving thorazine, as necessary, without either a signed doctor's order or any notation in the record of a telephone order." [15] The follow-up of the 1966 California audit released August 26, 1970, reveals that 734 doses of medication were administered without any signed physicians' orders.[16] (These figures are based on a review of one month's medical records of 106 Medi-Cal patients at fourteen nursing homes.)

Justification offered by nursing homes for keeping patients drugged is predictable: "The owner of one home in Los Angeles told me the first thing she does when a patient comes in the door is to give him a dose of Mellaril to calm his fright and make him feel at home." [17] When GAO auditors reviewed records relating to thirty-six California welfare patients selected at random in twelve nursing homes, they found that "approximately 50 percent of the patients were receiving sedatives during daylight hours. We were informed by nursing home personnel that sedatives were administered to patients with neurotic symtoms during daylight hours in order to level out their moods and keep them under control." [18] Dr. George Pennebaker of the California Department of Health Care Services sums up the choice nursing homes make daily: "The question arises of whether you're treating the patient or treating the staff. The patient who is not sedated requires more staff time." [19]

DRUG EXPERIMENTS

Drug companies frequently carry out experimental research on nursing home patients. One woman's report of an experiment involving her mother is a striking example of abuses that can occur. The case is unusual only in that the patient's family made exhaustive inquiries following her death and found that no one—not the government, nor the attending physician, nor the home—had been adequately protecting the patient.

According to a Food and Drug Administration report made at the family's insistence after the death of the patient, the G. D. Searle & Company had gained FDA permission to test "Anavar," a drug supposed to increase appetite and retard bone deterioration. The drug was already approved for use in doses of 2.5 milligrams two to four times a day for no more than three months. Searle wanted to test its usage over a long period of time at doses of 10 milligrams once a day.

Although the woman's daughter had expressly told the attending physician not to allow her mother to be given experimental drugs, the nursing home and attending physician approved her, among others, for the experiment.

After taking the drug for about six months, the patient became critically ill. Medical diagnoses never confirmed the cause of the illness. No move was made to find out whether the experimental drug had caused or contributed to the illness, and the drug continued to be given.

Two months later, the woman died. Both the home and the coroner who filled out the death certificate refused to tell the family exactly how or why the woman died. The home has refused to release the woman's medical records to her family.

The family did obtain a record of the drugs given and discovered that the patient had been taking an experimental drug. When they demanded to know why they had not been consulted, the home produced a "consent" document marked with the patient's X. Although the patient had been judged senile by her doctor, who recommended that she live in an institution, the home maintained and the FDA concurred that the "consent" of a person medically diagnosed as senile was sufficient.

The family further discovered that the woman's doctor believed the drug had been given as already approved and not as an experimental drug. He therefore made no attempt to see whether the drug was having ill effects. According to the daughter, because of certain allergies and an edema condition, it was possible that the drug had been highly dangerous for her mother.

This is a classic example of what can—and does— happen to unsuspecting nursing home patients. If "consent" can be obtained from a woman who has been diagnosed senile and confined to an institution for three years, it is meaningless. If a drug experiment can be carried out without the knowledge of the attending physician, medical protection is nonexistent. If nursing homes can refuse to release medical records to the patients' families, and if questionable deaths can go uninvestigated, protection is not being provided by those responsible. The Food and Drug Administration has been remiss in insuring protection through rigid requirements dealing with consent from responsible persons. The FDA is also responsible for guaranteeing medical surveillance and preventing harmful experiments.

DRUG KICKBACKS

Senator Ribicoff: Doctor, I am just curious. Is it fair to assume that kickbacks in the pharmaceutical field is a very widespread practice?

Dr. Apple: Well, Senator Ribicoff, with regard to the nursing home situation, it is one of the worst we have experienced in the history of our profession. It has been virtually a gun to the head of the pharmacist—you will not get in the door without a kickback.[20]

Drugs for nursing home patients can be obtained in a variety of ways. Paradoxically, the arrangement from which the patient stands to benefit most—dealing with a single pharmacist—is also the one with built-in possibilities for corruption. Some patients give their prescriptions to a friend or relative who takes it to be filled. However, because such autonomy gives a home no control over medications and because many patients seldom have visitors, a home may require that it provide all medications. Deplorably, only Vermont, Georgia, South Carolina, and Montana require contractual services if there is no pharmacy in the home.[21] Medicare is more rigid in requiring that the Extended Care Facility provide for obtaining drugs: "If the facility does not have a pharmacy department, it has provision for promptly and conveniently obtaining required drugs and biologicals from community pharmacies."[22] Some homes get their medications from several pharmacies; others use a single community pharmacist.

Dr. William S. Apple, Executive Director of the American Pharmaceutical Association, outlines the advantages to the patient of a home's dealing with one pharmacist:

After considerable study of this matter, we decided that the nursing home could best be served by having one pharmacy consultant aware of the complete operation of the nursing home, the staff that is available to them, the methods that are used to dispense the drugs to those patients, and preferably to obtain the drugs from one particular source—that is, one particular pharmacy—on a regular, routine basis. We find that this is the most economical system to arrange for the delivery of, the dispensing, the supervision and utilization of drugs in a nursing home or extended care facility. In other words, if we had 50 different pharmacies delivering 50 different prescriptions to a given nursing home every few days, I think we would have considerably more cost in the handling of the drugs inside the nursing homes and other problems that are generated by the need to control the drugs actually given to the patient on a daily basis.[23]

Competition among pharmacists to provide medicine and service to a nursing home gives the home the opportunity to shop around for the greatest benefits to the patient, or, in some cases, the greatest kickback for itself. Some kickback arrangements are simple: a pharmacist might give an owner or administrator a straight gift,[24] let him use his cottage at the beach,[25] or pay three thousand dollars monthly rent for an on-site pharmacy.[26] The kickback issue is complicated by the fact that nursing homes may provide pharmacists with a variety of bookkeeping services as well as its business. A pharmacist has to submit only one bill, not fifty or two hundred and fifty. He is, perhaps, assured prompt payment.[27] The nursing home, not the pharmacist, must collect the bills and take a loss on any that are not paid.

Central to the controversy is the percentage of the total bill which the pharmacist pays the nursing home for bookkeeping and for its business. It is the percentage of reduction from the total bill, not the reduction itself, which determines whether a nursing home is demanding a legitimate discount or a kickback.

In an article in *Modern Nursing Home,* Washington attorney Melvin O. Moehle casually assumes that "For the bookkeeping service and collection guarantee the pharmacy pays the nursing home a percentage (usually 15 to 25 percent) which is ordinarily a 'deduction' from

.the total bill." [28] Moehle's article—"Pharmacy Discounts: Illegal? Unethical? Dishonest?"—contains some other equally remarkable assertions. He admits that actual kickbacks, as opposed to "deductions," do exist. "This is not to say that there are not cases where kickbacks occur." He implies that those who might disagree with him on the discount rate also disagree with him on discounts in general, which they do not: "To blanket all pharmacy discounts as kickbacks is unfair and ignores the practice of granting discounts by both government and industry." Finally, Mr. Moehle's subtitle is deliberately misleading about the real issues he is discussing: "If legitimate service is provided, proper accounting procedures are used, and these guidelines are followed, pharmacy discounts should not be misunderstood." At stake is not service or guidelines but a percentage figure.

The American Pharmaceutical Association disagrees with Moehle. Its position was stated in a letter by Dr. Apple, published in *The APHA Newsletter:*

> Commercial charge account services, which provide pharmacists with the same services Mr. Moehle discusses, when provided by nursing homes, charge the pharmacist only from 7 to 12 percent of gross income. These commercial charge services realize what they regard as a reasonable profit from their services and charges. Nursing homes are ostensibly in the business of providing health care, not billing, and guarantee services for their suppliers. Pharmacists and other suppliers to nursing homes should not be required to reimburse nursing homes and related facilities for more than the reasonable costs of the services they are provided by the facility. Certainly, a flat percentage payment unrelated to cost and ranging from 15 to 25 percent is both exorbitant and unconscionable. [29]

Moehle defines "kickback" only as the simple cash kickback or favor: "Where the dollar goes in some individual's pocket for business favors given rather than to offset the legitimate cost of a business expense, it is a kickback." [30] That the high discount rate, not the cash sum or the house at the beach, is what nursing homes want from pharmacists is clear from the following cases.

In some cases, patients are subject to delays in receiving emergency drugs because of a percentage rate. In other cases, they merely have to pay more. "Some pharmacists have confided to me that they have to charge more than usual in order to give the large rebate," said Don L. McLeod, instructor in clinical pharmacy and director of the clinical and institutional extension program of the School of Pharmacy at the University of North Carolina.[31]

Joseph A. Pollak, an Ohio pharmacist, refused to allow a nursing home a 25 per cent discount; the home now uses a pharmacy 110 miles away, which could not even if willing, offer satisfactory emergency delivery of drugs.

> From 1959 to 1970 I had the privilege of servicing our local Nursing Home with prescription service as well as other commodities requested by patients as well as the operators. If need be, we made three to four trips (distance two miles) to satisfy their needs; this we did not mind because the prompt on the spot delivery was made as an appreciation of the business. On October 1, 1969, new operators took over and immediately they approached me—that unless I agreed to a 25% "kick-back" they would change. They did; however, they are now being serviced by a pharmacy located a distance of 110 miles. This is accomplished by Parcel Post.[32]

A major drug chain known for its low prices "no longer serves a single nursing home" because of the 15–20 per cent discount they were asked for. "Their dollar profit is greater than ours." The executive director of a midwestern state pharmaceutical association, in a telephone interview with a task force member, estimated that 40 per cent of the nursing homes served by pharmacists have an unrealistic service fee.

A pharmacist in the Fox River Valley in Wisconsin told us that he offered to pay a 22 per cent discount fee to a nursing home—2 per cent more than anyone else —but he was expected to make an additional under-the-table cash outlay every month. He says that the pharmacist now serving the home gives patients a seven- to fourteen-day supply of medicine twice a month and doubles the two dollar fee per prescription.

Both the pharmacist and the nursing home make more money.

Dr. Apple's testimony includes a letter describing the experience of still another pharmacist:

> I have just lost the nursing home that I have been the consultant for, for the last six years since I will not pay a 15 percent kickback as I was told I must by the minister who is the administrator of this church-owned home. I am finding out much to my dismay that pharmacy might be a profession, but there are very few if any professionals in it. We have two large homes in our town that are completely sewed up by an ex-member of our state board of pharmacy through a percentage kickback arrangement. Nice deal, huh? I am 35 years old, out of Pharmacy School for 14 years and have owned my own professional shop for eight years and I believe the long haired kids are about right. The Establishment is a bunch of crap. Professionalism will never get off the ground in pharmacy as long as we have to put up with the dollarhoos, discount merchants, and phyrocracy that we have in this town and state.[33]

The costs to the patient in terms of pharmaceutical service and money are incalculable. The costs to the Federal and state governments of high discounts can be estimated; the overall cost of pharmaceuticals in the Medical programs is about four hundred million dollars a year. Senator Ribicoff estimated that if all pharmacists are charged 20 per cent, those discounts would be eighty million dollars.[34] Dr. Apple said, "Very obviously, if a man has to pay a kickback, he is adding that to the bill so he can make a fair profit." [35]

In these three areas of misuse of prescribed drugs, unwarranted use of experimental drugs, and drug kickbacks, the nursing home industry has flagrantly abused the public interest. The dollar cost of drug abuse in nursing homes cannot be calculated, but certainly the aged and the government lose staggering sums because of the collusion between nursing homes and pharmacists, as druggists hike prices to make up for the kickbacks nursing homes force upon them. However, the most important toll is taken from the patients, who are the direct victims of irresponsible administration of drugs, unchecked prescriptions, unauthorized drug experiments, and the widespread practice of administering tranquilizers to keep the patients quiet. Not every nursing home is guilty of these abuses, but all the evidence indicates that they are widespread. As long as a nursing home staff maintains that its convenience is more important than the patients' health, and as long as HEW and the FDA continue to shun enforcement of important regulations, lives will be endangered by irresponsible drug administration.

THE INCENTIVE TO LIVE

A good home should have as its prime objective to preserve social and intellectual skills, as well as bodily well-being.[1]

Mr. P. was hospitalized with a stroke; he no longer needs intensive hospital treatment but he does need intensive nursing care. He is seventy-six years old and has been badly shaken by his illness and by the prospect of never returning to a full and useful life. All he really wants is to go home. But he must have care, someone to see that he gets the proper medication, someone to help him with the daily personal tasks he can no longer do for himself. He goes to a nursing home.

A nurse takes him to his room and as she is smoothing the sheets on the bed, she tells him that he will be in bed only for a few days. Then he will be able to get up, she says, and goes on to tell him about the activities at the home. Mr. P.'s only thought had been that he might never get out of bed. The nurse leaves, and Mr. P. begins to think about his own home and his illness. As his depression deepens, an aide brings in his dinner tray. The food is hot and looks good, though Mr. P. cannot eat much. The aide stays to talk for a few minutes and says that soon Mr. P. will be going downstairs for dinner. A nurse comes in later and asks how he liked his meal. Mr. P. tells her he likes more salt on his food. He is very tired, but as he drifts off to sleep he thinks that perhaps they are right, perhaps he will get out of bed again.

When Mr. R. arrives at the *** nursing home, he is

placed in a wheelchair and taken to what the staff member says is his room. Mr. R. is blind and has come to this home, he believes, to live until he dies. No one shows him his bed, or the bathroom, or how to signal for the nurse. Mr. R. does not know how long he sits in the wheelchair. An aide brings a dinner tray and goes away again; no one mentions eating in the dining room, and anyway Mr. R. cannot eat much. There is nothing to do except to wonder when someone will come. Soon the thought is consuming him: when will someone come?

Both of these situations were observed in different nursing homes. They have nothing to do with whether the patients get their medicine or their meals on time, or whether they are kept clean and safe. They have everything to do with whether Mr. P. will return to some form of active life, or whether Mr. R. will become increasingly withdrawn, increasingly depressed until life becomes a matter of waiting for death.

No matter how adequate the nursing care, what is all too often lacking in the nursing home is the incentive to get well. Only the few most expensive or well-endowed sectarian homes provide a conducive environment. As Dr. Sterling Brinkley, an HEW consultant, put it, "Kindness costs money in a nursing home." Our observations have led us to the conclusion that even when a patient's health needs are met, his emotional problems and social needs are often neglected. These needs are perhaps the most difficult of all the problems in caring for the aged; the most strictly enforced government regulations cannot insure kindness. But there are ways in which those who are responsible for care for the elderly, from Congressmen to community leaders, can help create a nursing home environment that is meaningful as well as therapeutic.

Training of nursing home personnel to meet the emotional and social needs of the patients is woefully lacking; in particular, aides get little instruction of any kind. Yet it is as important for the aides to know how to deal with an emotionally distressed patient as to know how to turn a patient properly in bed. Indeed, the high turnover rate for nursing home personnel may be traced not only to low wages and hard work but also to the stresses from dealing with aged people who may appear eccentric and cantankerous, overly demanding of time and understanding.

It is loneliness that makes a patient constantly ring for the nurse for company; it is often extremely irritating, especially to the staff member who has little understanding of an older person's desperate need for human contact. As one aide wrote, "I'm sick of the silent eyes of old people who have no one left; forced to die in a place that has no regard for their dignity or worth as human beings. . . . If we have the means to keep them alive, we have the means to allow them to live a meaningful old age." [2]

An understanding of what aging means is basic to adequate physical and emotional health care. Health problems of the elderly are often not related to one particular disease; old age makes the individual susceptible to many diseases. A simple cold can have serious effects on one's whole state of well-being. The aged are frequently unable to formulate symptomatic complaints and descriptions, thus heightening the deep-seated fear and anxiety that may have caused the physical symptoms in the first place. In such situations, mere custodial care is far from adequate. Those who care for the aged must feel for each patient and understand his idiosyncracies.

Many older people are naturally concerned with facing death. The staff must know how to deal with these anxieties when they occur, providing the sympathy each patient needs in response to his own fears. This natural fear may be hideously increased in nursing homes without a sensitivity to the problem:

> One day while I was visiting my mother, a poor soul had evidently passed away. The undertaker (I question that) arrived with a canvas bag. I presume the old soul had nobody at all. He talked for a bit with the head nurse, then went to the back of the building to get the lady. I heard a funny dragging [sound] and looked up to see him pulling the bag (now full) down the home's at least 80 cement and wooden steps. I have never seen such a thing or ever want to again. The reaction on the faces of the old folks was rather shocking. They probably pictured themselves going like that. [3]

In one nursing home we visited, the phone number for the funeral home was prominently posted at the nursing station in the hall, and the patients walked past it every day. Still another home was located immediately adjacent to a cemetery and funeral home.

A common problem in nursing homes is what one gerontologist calls "infantilism," the tendency to treat the elderly as children instead of as mature adults suffering from ill health or the natural processes of aging. We encountered numerous examples of infantilism:

> Two of us went to visit a nursing home, and the head nurse was showing us around. She took us into a room and smiled brightly at the residents and said, "Good morning, ladies." Then in a voice just a wee bit softer, she proceeded to tell us all about each patient. I'm sure they could hear her even if they were deaf—you never can tell how much a deaf person can hear. In another room, she went up to a man and said jokingly, "Oh, Mr. X., I hear you've wet yourself already." Mr. X. looked humiliated and saddened.[4]

Dr. Robert N. Butler, Washington, D.C., psychiatrist and gerontologist, said that this reaction to infantilism stems from the fact that helplessness breeds patronizing.[5] Furthermore, a staff member who himself fears growing older and dying may try to remove himself from an anxiety-producing situation by treating the aged person as a child.

The nursing home staff is often patronizing. Many aged people are incontinent; the phrase, "Oh, Mrs. Y., you've wet your bed again!" is heard time and again in nursing homes. Mrs. Y., who may have perfectly good sense, is naturally humiliated. As a result, her reaction may be to do less and less for herself, to become more helpless and childish than is necessary. The best approach is for the nurse to encourage Mrs. Y. to learn the use of a bedpan; a physical therapist may be able to teach her how to get out of bed and use the facilities.

In our interview with Dr. Butler, he made a statement that may be surprising: "There is no such thing as senility." He added that senility is a word much overused and little understood. Cerebral arteriosclerosis is the medical term for a condition that means that the flow of blood to the brain is impeded by hardening of the arteries, making the individual forgetful and confused. A common symptom of this condition is a return to childhood memories, which Dr. Butler calls "life review." He believes that many elderly people try to understand their lives by reviewing what they have done. If hardening of the arteries occurs, they remain in the time period they were reviewing at that point. Thus many aged people can be perfectly normal one day and be talking about going to see their long-dead mother the next. Dr. Butler also suggests that elderly people may be excessively irritable because they are preoccupied with "life review" and coping with feelings of guilt that may arise.

Reviewing one's life is an experience common to almost everyone, Dr. Butler says, but it seems to intensify among the aged. This may explain the sense of aloofness of an older person, and the impression that he is "off in his own world." The nature of reviewing one's life is both conscious and unconscious; its basis is the sense of impending death, its function is "reintegration of personality and preparedness for death." It offers an explanation for increased reminiscence, disturbed behavior such as depression and despair, and positive behavioral traits common among the aged such as candor, serenity, and wisdom. Psychiatrists believe that the life review process is triggered by the sense of approaching dissolution and death, stirred by current isolated incidents and experiences. Too often people regard the reminiscing of the aged as a symptom of "senility."

None of this is to suggest that the elderly do not suffer from mental illness. They do, and in considerable numbers, but a study made by the Institute of Mental Health points out that the mental illnesses of the aged are much the same as those of the younger population, "unrelated to either cerebral vascular disease or age." [6] Unfortunately, as Dr. Butler said, elderly patients suffering from the same mental sicknesses as the young are generally regarded as untreatable, passed over as simply "senile," and put away to vegetate. Forty per cent of the psychiatrists in this country treat no patient over the age of fifty-five, and only 1 per cent have extensive contact with the aged, according to one study. [7] In the U.S. there are very few diagnostic or active psychotherapeutic centers for geriatric patients.

Thus nursing homes are often required to cope with patients with as great a variety of mental and emotional stability as exists in the broader population. All too often, however, the aged are lumped together in a group labeled "senile." Their individual disorders are denied the specific psychiatric or other treatment they require. Mentally healthy older persons are often treated as senile because of health problems, such as incontinence, or normal characteristics of aging, such as "life review." If the nursing home personnel understood what aging means, how it is like and unlike other stages of maturity, it might help them overcome the impatience and despair that is all too prevalent in a nursing home.

Active involvement in life is as vital to a patient's emotional well-being as proper medication is to his physical health. Yet in many homes patients are regularly placed in front of the television set in lieu of activities that could give them an incentive to become more independent. Often they are simply left in bed. Coordinating patient activities is an important area that is sorely neglected in many nursing homes.

On Sunday, July 19, 1970, St. Joseph's Manor had only one patient in bed, and that was due to the fact that the patient needed oxygen. (It was expected that she, too, would soon be out of bed.) Indeed, St. Joseph's Manor was alive with activity. The pleasant lawn is full of benches and shrines on which residents sit and talk. Their greenhouse provides all the flowers for the Manor. One of their residents, a distinguished artist, has equipped an art studio and teaches other residents how to paint. Children from the town also come for instruction. The home provides well-equipped occupational and physical therapy rooms, not to mention a beautiful auditorium. The home has a special bus with an hydraulic lift to raise wheelchairs into the bus. The residents take trips to the beach, the local shopping center, New York City, and they often go on picnics.

In a nursing home in Virginia, nearly one-half of the patients were confined to their beds. One blind woman we got to know in this home could walk with assistance and could certainly sit in a wheelchair, but she lay in bed all day and had bedsores as big as a fist.

In the * * * home, there were almost no activities. On warm days, the patients were wheeled up to the front porch where they were able to watch the cars rush by on a dirty highway, or overlook the adjacent cemetery. A few watched an unfocused television, while others sat around the nurses' station and stared absently at the opening and shutting of the elevator door. There were no newspapers, magazines, or books in evidence and rarely any planned activities. Once a week, a cart was brought around from the local drugstore and the patients were able to pay exorbitant prices to buy a few items to brighten up their day. Immediately after dinner, the patients started asking the nurses if they could go to bed; they had nothing else to do.[8]

In many homes we observed patients gathered in the lounge waiting for dinner an hour or more before the meal time. They would sit in the auditorium waiting for a movie more than an hour before the film was scheduled to begin. The home did not even have to post the name of the film; they simply announced that a film would be shown, knowing that patients would be all too glad for any amusement to break the monotony of their day.

Television—focused or unfocused—plays an important part in the lives of most nursing home patients. In many homes, the aged are systematically gotten out of bed, dressed, fed, and placed in front of the television until a nurse comes to get them again. Even the blind are placed in front of the television to soak in the daily soap operas. Many nursing homes appear to find an investment in a color TV cheaper than paying for an activities program, so the television continues to take the place of more constructive activities.

An activities program, however, can be an essential part of nursing home life. An older man had said very little since entering the home some months earlier. One day the activities director showed a film on gardening. In the discussion period that followed, the man could not stop talking about his own garden. Properly operated, the activities program can function as the primary stimulus for the individuality every patient brings to the nursing home and all too often loses there. Once individual interests are expressed, the nursing home should provide an outlet for them—in this case, a garden for the older man, who could also teach other patients the skills of gardening.[9]

The activities program is coordinated with the occupational therapy program in the best nursing homes. Rugs and knitted items made in occupational therapy sessions may be sold at a community bazaar, a good way to create community within the home and draw in the community outside. Many gerontologists feel that even the most confused and disturbed older person can be involved in activities.

Some of the entertainment and recreation, encompassing a broad range of interests and abilities, that a nursing home can provide include the following:

carving	movies
ceramics	museum trips
church attendance	painting
cooking	parties and gatherings
crafts	puzzles
do-it-yourself books	radios
games	records
greenhouses	sewing
grounds to walk and tend	shopping excursions
indoor exercise room	singing
knitting	television
library	visiting other patients
magazines	weaving

Although visitors are encouraged at most nursing homes, in a study of ten personal care homes in West Virginia, only 60 per cent of the patients received regular visitors. (A regular visitor is considered one who comes once a week.) The other 40 per cent had a visit once a month or less, including "gang visits" by church groups, school glee clubs, and service organizations.[10]

Homes can encourage regular visitors to help with activities that include all the patients. The Mary Manning Walsh Home run by the Carmelite Sisters in New York City has an organization composed of patients' relatives who arrange parties and entertainment, planning some activity at least one night a week. A son or daughter may work the home switchboard once a week while talking to his or her parent. The parent begins to feel that the nursing home is his home when his children accept it as such and come to visit as regularly as they would in his own home.

Religion is an important part in the lives of many older people. Many newer homes have chapels that offer services as often as once a day. If medically possible, nursing home residents should be encouraged to attend local churches. Churchgoing is an excellent way to involve patients in the broader community beyond the walls of the nursing home. Church groups as well as local service clubs can also play a part in the life of the nursing home. Many residents are able to attend meetings outside the home; these community groups should not neglect nursing home residents who are able to join them. The more ties the nursing home develops with the community, the more incentive their patients have to become involved in a meaningful life. For example, transportation to the polls on election day should be provided, or arrangements made for residents to vote by absentee ballot. There are a myriad of ties the nursing home can develop between its patients and the surrounding community, a community to which the nursing home patient often can and should be a contributing part.

But all this costs money. Our visits to a random sampling of twenty nursing homes suggested that few have adequate incentive programs. Of the twenty we visited, only St. Joseph's Manor in Connecticut appeared to offer an environment where elderly people lived meaningful, full, and productive lives.[11] One indication that nursing homes are often neglecting the emotional and social needs of the elderly is the fact that the major deficiency in homes certified for Medicare is the lack of an adequate social services program. Over 30 per cent of the nursing homes certified for Medicare today have deficiencies in this area.[12] Medicare standards require that "there is a designated member of the staff of the facility who will take responsibility, when medically related social problems are recognized, for action necessary to solve them." The standards say that this person may be a full-time or part-time social worker employed by the facility or a person on the staff "who is suited by training and/or experience in related fields to find community resources to deal with the social problems." If the facility does not have a social worker on its staff, there must be "an effective arrangement with a public or private agency, which may include the local welfare department, to provide social service consultation." [13]

The social service staff member should also be responsible for training other employees to "understand emotional problems and social needs of sick and infirm aged persons," to recognize social problems of patients and the means of taking appropriate action to solve them. The standards further specify that "social and emotional factors related to the patient's illness, to his response to treatment, and to his adjustment to care in the facility [should be] recognized and appropriate action . . . taken when necessary to obtain casework services to assist in resolving problems in these areas." [14]

Social services cover a wide range of patient needs, including his financial situation and coordination of the various assistance programs for which he may qualify. Social services also include family problems, and problems related to the patient's adjustment to the nursing home. The nursing home with a full-fledged social services program is generally more attuned to meeting patient needs—whether they be occupational therapy, activities, community involvement, or obtaining a piece of furniture from the patient's former home, or arranging for a volunteer to visit a patient without a family. Nurses and aides can fulfill these needs only in the most haphazard fashion, particularly if they are not trained, or have not been taught to recognize them in the first place.

The social worker can also become a way for the patient to influence how the nursing home is run. In almost all homes, decisions about activities and care are made by the staff; the patient has little opportunity to affect these decisions. As Dr. Robert Butler told us, "Institutions are built more for themselves than for the individuals." [15] The social services staff can be the means for accommodating the institution to the patient. Our letters and observations indicate that adjustment to a nursing home generally means that the patient gives up his desires and often his individuality, to meet the institutional demands.

Family problems also fall within the province of the social worker. A nurse in a nursing home wrote us, "I hope something can be done to make these old people more comfortable. A lot of sons and daughters bring their parents to us and then never come to see them again." [16] The social worker can bring comfort to the patient by working with families to help them cope with the feelings that led them to place their parent in a nursing home.

Attention to personal problems is often a luxury for the elderly in a nursing home, not because it is inessential, but because it is so rare. Certainly medical and nursing care, food, and safety precautions are basic to providing for the welfare of the nursing home resident. The remaining problem is to make life worth living to the older person, infirm, often ill, perhaps cut off from his former active life, his family and friends. In some cases, denial of these needs is equal to denial of food as far as the patient's health is concerned.

4 Outside the Nursing Home

PROBLEMS OF AMERICA'S AGED

In 1969, the American people spent five billion dollars on preparations to keep them looking young [1]; in 1970, the Federal government spent one and a third billion dollars on Old Age Assistance.[2] The comparative statistics summarize neatly the problem of the old in the United States.

Why and how the cult of youth developed in America —whether the cause is to be sought in the collective memory of frontier days, in the relative youth of the nation itself, in regret for the loss of our national innocence—is not of particular significance here. What is important is that, in our single-minded pursuit of youth, we have systematically ignored those who are old. The American Indians stood in the path of what we conceived to be our national destiny, so we shoved them by the way; we have done the same with the old, who, like the Indians and the blacks, are an oppressed minority; we have segregated them from the rest of society.

It was not always so, and it need not be so now. Time was, in rural America especially, that children, parents, grandparents, and sometimes great-grandparents lived under the same roof. This is still the typical structure of families in Italy. But modern Americans, taking a cue from their grandfathers' treatment of the Indians, have packed the aged off to reservations—to nursing homes and "senior villages" in Florida.

If an old man or woman dares to stay in society with the rest of us, we do our best to make his short time miserable. In most cases, we force him to leave his job simply because he passes the magic age of sixty-five. We replace his independent livelihood with pitifully small Social Security or welfare benefits. If he tries to take a job, we discriminate against him; if he somehow manages to find a job, we take away the Social Security benefits he has paid for all his life. If he is disabled, or weak, or simply in need of a little help now and again, we offer him next to nothing in the way of home care services, at any price. He must go to a nursing home.

It is too often a fault of American approaches to problem-solving that, instead of exploiting and increasing the flexibility of the programs we have, we create endless new ones. There are six Federal agencies that deal with the aged; the fragmentation of services has become so grave that a new agency has been proposed whose sole function would be to coordinate the activities of the others. Ironically, however, the result of this fragmentation has not been to increase the number of approaches to the health and social care of the aged but to limit them rigidly to institutional care. The practical alternatives for an aged person in need of limited care are a paltry three: hospitalization, institutionalization in a nursing home, or life with younger, more capable relatives. Life at home, except for the few lucky or rich enough to snare one of the few available nurses or homemakers, is impossible. Medicare will pay for one hundred visits a year by home health aides, but only one out of seven Medicare recipients lives in an area where such services can be obtained.

About 25 per cent of the elderly in this country live alone or with nonrelatives. For these five million people, life is a daily bout with an income that may once have been sufficient, with tasks that once were simple, with an unfamiliar and unfriendly loneliness. Going to the grocery store can be a major undertaking as the older person struggles with inadequate transportation, fear (many of the victims of street crime are over sixty-five), and the difficulty of lugging home large, cumbersome bags of groceries, only to cook and eat alone. The result is that thousands of older people have serious health problems due to deficient diets. They do not need a nursing home —and the already crowded nursing homes do not need them—but for many the nursing home is the only alternative.

The right to live outside a nursing home is surely as precious as the right to good care inside one, yet it is astonishingly difficult for millions of elderly people to maintain a decent life on their own. The first problem of the aged in their struggle to live independently is money. Some seven million older people, more than one-third of the over-sixty-five population, are impoverished and must depend on someone else—their families or government—for income assistance. The average Social Security payment to a couple retiring in 1950 met half the budget cost estimated by the U.S. Bureau of Labor Statistics as necessary for self-support; today it meets less than one-third.[3] In urban areas, the percentage of living costs covered by Social Security is even lower; BLS budget estimates for a retired couple to live "comfortably but not luxuriously" in autumn, 1968, were $3,869 a year; for a single retired person, $2,000. Projections to 1980 indicate that more than two-thirds of all retired couples will receive less than $3,000 annually in Social Security benefits. According to an administrator of the city's Office for the Aging, in New York City in 1970, the average income of persons over sixty-five was $1,500—less than four dollars a day. The mayor of Malden, Massachusetts, told a state hearing that he had seen aged people go into a restaurant, order a cup of hot water, and pour in ketchup to make tomato soup —a trick learned back in the Depression.

Social Security benefits are not the only kind of income assistance. Some 2,050,000 elderly people receive public assistance payments under Old Age Assistance. OAA funds are dispensed to the states on a matching basis, so that the poorer states give lower benefits. In South Carolina the payment is $48.70 a month; in New York, $93.60; in New Hampshire, $168.10. The national average payment is $75.45 a month, about $900 per year, and certainly not enough for subsistence.⁴ Medicare and Medicaid now help to pay the medical expenses of older people, which are nearly three times larger than those of the young, but these programs either do not cover all medical costs, or cover them only for limited times or up to a certain point. Medical costs continue to fall heaviest on those least able to pay them.

Beyond their financial needs, denial of services and opportunities may prevent elderly people from living full lives in the community. They have special housing, transportation, and social needs that are often not available even if the aged could afford them, although again money is generally at the root of these troubles. As Commissioner John B. Martin of the Administration on Aging has said,

> Older Americans have been expected to be content with half measures—discounts, tax concessions, reduced bus fares, and charity from their children or volunteer agencies. They have watched as the special needs of other segments of the population are rightfully understood and met, while their own special needs for mobility, for increased socialization, for the sense of worth which comes from productive capacity, go unheeded.⁵

A psychiatrist who specializes in problems of the aging has said that "one-third of older Americans are living in quiet despair, stemming both from physical and spiritual poverty that in turn stems from the chilling realization of powerlessness and non-participation." ⁶

Unlike other segments of society, the elderly have formed a coherent political force only rarely, as in the Johnson-Goldwater election of 1964. Although older Americans make up 15 to 17 per cent of the voters, they almost never vote as a bloc and have few effective political organizations to voice their special needs. Since their needs are rarely formulated as political issues, many social and poverty programs that benefit other groups omit the elderly entirely.

The drawbacks to the poverty programs dealing with the elderly are indicative of larger problems. An official in the Human Resources Office of Washington's District government said that when poverty funds are cut, programs for the elderly are usually the first to go. When it is a choice between a program for the elderly and a program like Headstart for children, the tendency is to give the money to the children's program. The point is not that Headstart should not have the money but that both needs should be met and that if the nation were as concerned about its aged as it is about its deprived young (and if the aged formed a political group), both needs would be met.

Gerontologist Dr. Robert Butler describes older people as victims of "age-ism." Age-ism means that a great many older people are "segregated" and pushed off into "retirement communities" and "housing for the elderly." Age-ism means "only 3 per cent of the research budget of the National Institute of Mental Health is spent in relevant research on aging, and less than 1 per cent of the budget of the entire National Institutes of Health is devoted to the study of aging phenomena," while 25 per cent of the public mental hospital admissions are people sixty-five and older. Age-ism is the result of "the stereotype of the undeserving." [7]

HOUSING

When programs are formed for the elderly, as Dr. Butler points out, they are usually "segregated" programs of housing or other services. Low-income housing, for example, is a special need of the elderly who are likely to have taken severe income cuts upon retiring and frequently cannot afford the rents they paid when working. According to an HEW official, some two to five million of the twelve million households of older people would like specially designed housing. Every senior housing development has a waiting list, not because older people like to live apart from other age groups, but because so little low-income housing is available in society at large. One Maryland housing development, planned originally for older people only, could not fill its units and had to open to adults of all ages. While this is unusual, it indicates that when people have a choice, they resist being segregated in housing.

Urban renewal programs often cover areas in which one-half or one-third of the population is made up of older people, most of whom are displaced when the bulldozers move in. The Model Cities program could give special attention to the needs of the aged. Low-rent housing for the elderly—with such features as easy-to-open windows, and kitchens and baths that require little stooping—should no longer be built in isolated communities designed just for the aged; it should be integrated into the wider community, for the benefit of both the aged and the young. The Model Cities program should also provide funds to improve public transportation systems by making them more economical and safer.

Home repair services should also be available for older people who own their own homes. For most of the elderly, their home is their only major asset; two out of three own their own homes, and 80 per cent are free of mortgages. Half have sunk twenty-five thousand dollars or more into their homes, yet many are "house-poor" because of limited, fixed retirement incomes. Inflation and rising property taxes make it increasingly difficult for the elderly to hang on to the one asset they are likely to have.

For those who wish to sell their homes and live in smaller quarters, there are difficulties, particularly for those living alone. Anyone at all familiar with the housing problems in American cities knows that inexpensive housing—or even reasonably priced housing—is almost impossible to find except in unsafe or inconvenient locations. This problem is severe for widows and single women, who comprise well over one-quarter of the aged population. Six out of ten of all aged women living alone have incomes below the poverty line.

HOME CARE SERVICES

To remain in their own homes within the community, the elderly often need homemaker services. Many also require home health services, for which Medicare and Medicaid pay. However, the Social and Rehabilitation Service of HEW estimated in 1967 that only six thousand home health aides were available, although some two hundred thousand were needed and little is being done to increase the number. Some suggest a "new careers" component and on-the-job training for health aides built into the Medicare payment program. These aides could be trained as personal care workers and then proceed up the ladder of health care personnel, relieving the personnel shortage in nursing homes and hospitals as well as helping house-bound elderly people.

As an example of home care services offered by the community, let us look at the programs in Washington, D.C. There is one homemaker service in Washington, D.C.; most home care programs in the District area are health programs. There are the Visiting Nurses, which is privately run; the Georgetown Hospital home care program, which serves only twenty cancer patients at a time; and the D.C. General Hospital home care program. While home medical care is essential, the homemaker service, which provides help with daily essentials like shopping, cooking, and cleaning, is a necessary complement and one for which Medicare funds are not available. The D.C. Homemaker Service takes care of 426 older people; it has turned down 700 requests because of lack of staff. According to program officials, at least 500 of these rejected applicants were in pressing need of the Service, but inadequate financing, coupled with a shortage of social workers willing to work with the elderly, has limited the program.[8]

The D.C. General Hospital home care program covers medical needs such as nursing, medicine, physical and occupational therapy, and social work. Officials of this program realize that there is also a need for housekeeping services which, because of their limited facilities and funding, the program cannot provide. Many requests for housekeeping services have been turned down. As of August 10, 1970, the service had one medical director, nine private physicians (internists working half time), five full-time social workers, two half-time podiatrists, two physical therapists and a vacancy for a third, a vacancy for an occupational therapist, one speech therapist, one nutritionist, fourteen health aides, and nine people on the clerical staff. With these limited resources they are servicing 470 patients; 200 are in personal care homes and the rest are living in private homes. Most health aides have a background in practical nursing and generally give personal care. They cannot give medication but can handle simple nursing duties such as changing bandages under the supervision of a public health nurse.

One staff member said that the program tries to get patients out of the hospital and into their homes sooner, and to ease the shortage of hospital beds. But unless other hospitals become interested in this sort of program, and unless homemaker services expand, too many patients, especially older patients who could live at home if home care were generally available, will jam the District's hospitals.

Housekeeping services are available to welfare recipients if a doctor so recommends and if the recipient can find a housekeeper. Washington's Public Assistance will then pay two hundred dollars a month for the service. Staff in the home care program at D.C. Hospital feel these services should be expanded and help should be given in finding a housekeeper. They also stress the need for expanding other medical services, providing transportation to eye and dental clinics, for example, or adding eye and dental care to the home care program.

A number of conclusions can be drawn from Washington, D.C.'s failures to provide adequate noninstitutional care for its elderly residents. It is not enough that all the components of total care outside a hospital are available. (The District provides home medical and nursing care, housekeeping services through voluntary and Public Assistance organizations, and hospitals interested in working with the home care services.) The chief difficulties seem to be administrative and financial. As in the case of Federal nursing home programs, no one has the responsibility to develop a total home care and health policy for the Washington area. What programs there are were developed independently and operate fragmentedly; if they happen to work together at times, it is only a fortunate coincidence. Until the time comes when these disparate parts are joined into a whole, the aged will have to trust to luck.

OTHER COMMUNITY NEEDS

Suggestions have been made for comprehensive community centers, perhaps located in public housing developments, to coordinate all the needs of the elderly. A program proposed in New York included the following recommendations:

1. community-based geriatric centers to provide diagnosis, short-term treatment, and placement;
2. small residential units specializing in long-term care of mildly confused but ambulatory elderly persons;
3. expanded and broadened services of nursing home infirmary sections in city or county infirmaries, specialized sections of state mental hospitals, and homes for the aged;
4. expanded public housing to provide comprehensive services to elderly tenants;
5. state and mental hospitals with increased emphasis on geriatric psychotherapy;
6. legislation to provide for a "conservator" for the property of an older person during times when he may be temporarily unable to cope with his responsibilities.[9]

CAREER OPPORTUNITIES

The country is moving toward earlier retirement at the same time that the life expectancy of the population is increasing. Although the problems accompanying retirement have long been recognized, little has been done either to provide new opportunities for work after retirement or to prepare people for the period following an active career.

If current labor force participation trends continue, one out of every six men in the fifty-five to sixty-four age category will no longer be in the work force by the time he reaches his sixty-fourth birthday. Ten years ago this ratio was only one out of eight.

Psychiatrists point out that enforced retirement and the absence of social roles often affect the mental health

of those over sixty-five.[10] The incidence of psycho-
pathology rises with age, as do depression and suicide.
The suicide rate, in fact, is highest among white men
in their eighties. There is a large incidence of psychiatric disorders among nursing home residents. One
study estimates that 87 per cent of the patients suffer
from mental disorders.[11] One-quarter of all new admissions to public, state, county, and municipal mental hospitals are sixty-five and older.

The evidence clearly points to the need for psychiatry
to play a larger role in the health care of the elderly. Yet
the Joint Commission on Mental Illnesses and Health
does not have among its agencies a group concentrating on the mental problems of the aged, nor is there a
psychiatrist among its members. It has been proposed
that the Senate Subcommittee on Retirement and the
Individual establish a commission on mental health and
illnesses of the aging and retired.

The income difficulties and mental stress of retirement both require attention; often a single solution
takes care of both problems. Presently, an older person
under the age of seventy-two loses his Social Security
benefits—which he has earned through his Social Security taxes—if he earns more than $1,680 a year. He
is thereby penalized for working. Many people sixty-
five and over are capable of working but cannot get jobs.
Even in the case of disabled workers, 64 per cent are
employable in the competitive market with retraining.[12]
But very few training programs are oriented toward the
elderly. In one state, out of the 11,512 persons trained
in 1964, only 502 were fifty-five or over. In the same
state, 59,744 people fifty-five and over were seeking un-
employment insurance benefits. Even volunteer jobs are
limited for older people, although occupation in the
social services could be a productive and satisfying way
for a retired person to spend his time.

We need many more employment services especially
concerned with older people. One proposal is a computerized skills-matching register in each community
to serve as a clearing-house for jobs and services for the
elderly. This service could provide Federally sponsored
job training programs concentrated on older peoples'

needs. It could create additional employment opportunities by encouraging private, government, and voluntary agencies to employ older people.

A number of services in the Washington area function as free employment agencies for persons over sixty.[13] One is the Senior Citizens Employment Service in Alexandria, Virginia, which offers training in the Good Neighbor Family Aid Program for those whose skills and experience are in homemaking and a Senior Home Craftsman Program to train the elderly to do minor home repair work.

In 1969, this Service handled 387 requests from employers and 267 job applications, and made 140 placements. An employee of the agency reported that "there is usually more of a demand from workers than we can fill. . . . The need to be needed—aside from, or complementary to, financial need—brings many applicants to the service. . . . The problem of employer resistance, or reluctance of employers to consider over-60's as desirable employees, is a diminishing one." This agency spokesman said that "employers are becoming increasingly aware of the qualifications of the over-60's, with their dependability and wide range of experience." [14]

Despite some improvement, notably caused by the prohibition against age discrimination in the 1964 Civil Rights Act, the problems persist. Almost one-fifth of the aged work or want to work, but the temporary dislocations caused by the current economic slump aside, many cannot find jobs. Of the 1.1 million aged women in the labor force, over half are interested in full-time jobs and cannot get them.[15]

RURAL AREAS

The problems of the aged in rural areas are even more severe than those of the urban aged. One-third of the older population in rural areas is below the poverty line; the figure increases to one-half when those who have moved to the city are included. Most became poor as they became old; most are too proud for welfare, although one out of ten is eligible. Pension plans do not exist for those who earned their living in agriculture, and one can no longer farm without large amounts of credit.

The welfare system has been a total disaster in rural areas, in part because people are more accustomed to being self-sufficient. In urban areas, welfare involves indignities, but they are impersonal; in the country, anonymity disappears, and the fact that one is on welfare is embarrassing and degrading. Rural areas lack the trained social workers, health clinics, gerontologists, and mental hospitals that can be found in the cities. Accident rates are higher in rural areas than in cities, but the number of doctors is lower. Rural areas also lack social services and community action agencies; cities are higher on the priority list of money grants for poverty programs. Recreational activity is often nonexistent in small rural towns, where the migration of younger people to the cities has left a depressed economic situation. The major way to raise public funds is through property taxes, which hit the elderly hardest. Poverty programs are needed to help these people, yet rural aged poor are the lowest on the priority list.

One promising program, funded by the Labor Department and sponsored by the National Farmer's Union, is the Green Thumb/Green Light program. Green Thumb pays retired men up to sixteen hundred dollars a year for work on beautification projects. Perhaps its most spectacular success has been in Newton County, Tennessee, a small rural area of forty-eight hundred that had been left stranded when competition drove most of its farmers out of business. There was no public transportation and not even a first aid kit for miles around. Mail was delivered on horseback. The total county budget was $160,000. The biggest sources of personal income were Social Security benefits and welfare. The average resident was sixty years old, but the only Federal program in the area was a Neighborhood Youth Corps. When four Green Thumb organizers marched into Newton County, they became the largest employers in the county. They recruited a team which fixed up the road and roadside parks, hoping to make the area into a tourist attraction. Before anyone realized what was happening, Al Capp came along, bought some land, and created Dog Patch, U.S.A., a major tourist attraction. Now "Dogpatchers" and "Green Thumbers" have the largest payrolls in a prosperous community.[16]

The average new Green Thumb employee has been unemployed for four years; he has lost his friends, is lonely and aimless. Becoming a Green Thumber gives him a social role again. For the women in the community—and women outnumber men two to one—the Green Light program provides employment as teachers' aides and community service aides. Green Light employees also work in school kitchens, in libraries, with retarded children, for government agencies and food stamp centers. Health and beauty have blossomed in these people like a second youth; they have a reason to live again. Older people thrive with work, and in this unusual program they can pace themselves.

Project FIND (Friendless, Isolated, Needy, Disabled) began as a pilot "out-reach" project funded by the Office of Economic Opportunity to explore the problems of older people in urban areas. After its contract was up, FIND was picked up by some communities, among them New York City's West Side.

One of the biggest problems that Project FIND had to tackle was that caused by the eviction of elderly people from the hotels around Times Square, where there is a high concentration of people over sixty-five.[17] Following a Project FIND demonstration of some one hundred persons in Times Square on March 23, 1968, relocation help was brought to seventy-nine persons forced to evacuate the Hotel Flander and Rex on West 47th Street. There were one hundred forty living in the hotel at the time; seventy-nine were given direct assistance, including the use of a moving van and help from the Departments of Relocation and Social Services in finding a place to stay. Fifty-four of the seventy-nine were over the age of sixty, reported a FIND field worker.[18] The director of Project FIND says that

> this makes six hotels evacuated since last November [1968] with more than 500 senior citizens displaced. It's the same pattern: here this lady has lived in her hotel—and we don't want to say where yet—for thirty years, and she gets a letter notice that she must move. The hotel did not

advise her that she is covered by rent control and is entitled to a minimum of $450 to relocate and help in finding a place to live. She has nothing to worry about; they can't throw her out without a court order. But the others in the hotel are not protected and can be locked out of their rooms.[19]

The occasional successes of groups like Green Thumb/ Green Light and FIND are exceptions to an unfortunate rule. As if the psychological and economic stresses of encountering retirement were not enough, the aged must face it with only minimal assistance from Federal, state, and local authorities. The success of the Green Thumb program in Newton County, Tennessee, indicates how easily imaginative social action can change a declining community; the presence there of the Neighborhood Youth Corps indicates how easily a fragmented system of social services can misapply its energies. The struggles of FIND in New York City indicate how simply governmental agencies can work at cross-purposes. As poor as the quality of care received in nursing homes is, conditions outside the homes are little better than those within: the food is bad, medical care is hard to get, and, for far too many, there is nothing to do.

"Two kinds of people wait in the Port Authority Bus Terminal near Times Square. Some are waiting for buses. Others are waiting for death." [20] With these words, *The New York Times* of May 18, 1970, launched an account of how some two hundred to two hundred fifty retired people enjoy their leisure in a bus terminal. Why do they congregate there? One old man told the *Times* reporter that he came to Port Authority to avoid looking at the four walls of his one-room apartment.

"To old people whose dwellings are tiny or dreary or places of endless boredom, the waiting room is a kind of indoor park. It never rains in the Port Authority bus terminal. The overhead bulbs are as steady as the sun in a cloudless sky."

Once in a while the police scatter them, but the old people return in a matter of minutes. Port Authority officials view them as "a mild form of nuisance," and would like to construct a park nearby to attract some of the elderly sitters. Fortunately for Port Authority regulars, Project FIND is planning a coffee house for the aged in the area. In the meantime, FIND runs a table in the station to assist the elderly with such services as half-fare subway cards. Most of the "regulars," said one FIND official, are from the West Side of Manhattan, and "behave like solid members of the middle class, upper middle class at that." In her opinion, their greatest fears are placement in a nursing home or joining the welfare rolls.

The director of New York's West Side office for the aging said, "They feel that either [alternative] cancels them out as a person. They feel that this is the end of them. That is why they struggle so hard to stay independent, 'to be free,' as they put it."

SOLUTIONS IN OTHER COUNTRIES [1]

The aged can be free, if the United States will stop pouring all its money into dangerously inadequate institutions and start trying to keep the aged *out* of institutions. Great Britain, Denmark, and Sweden have gained reputations for having developed successful ways to care for their aged; common to all three is their emphasis on preventive medicine and home care. Their success is not complete; and because we have had to rely on government statements about health care, the picture we present here probably glosses over some serious problems. However, even if none of these countries measures up to its ideals of health care for the aged, they have at least a coherent set of ideals that they are struggling to make real. An exact comparison between the United States and any of these countries is impossible in the face of important social and economic differences. Yet a comparison is instructive, for it shows how a fully flexible program has been built, and, with allowances for national differences, could be built in the United States.

GREAT BRITAIN

In the United States, one of the many roadblocks to a successful program of preventive medicine has been the absence of a national health insurance program.

Because it costs from ten to twenty dollars just to visit the doctor for a checkup, the temptation is strong to stay away until disease strikes or becomes more severe. Thanks to the National Health Service, which was established in Great Britain in 1946, the incentive works the other way; for all its troubles (and they have, reportedly, been legion), the National Health Service has made the United Kingdom the envy of many Americans.

For the aged, preventive medicine has another dimension, too. The process of growing old is fraught with medical perils. The most expensive of these are so-called catastrophic illnesses—the health crisis that comes when an older person falls and breaks a hip, or has a heart attack, and needs intensive hospital care—and chronic illnesses, which require prolonged attention, though not necessarily in a hospital. The secret of the success of the British program is that it strives mightily to avoid putting the victims of chronic illness into a hospital or nursing home.

The theory is that older people should be assisted to remain independent of institutional care for as long as possible, and the theory is put into practice through extensive programs of community care. For those who cannot cook, cannot afford balanced meals, or cannot obtain housekeeping services, hot meals are served at centers throughout the country. The government pays for home nursing services and for housekeepers, both of which are easy to obtain. Home care is provided through the Crown's Health Visiting Services, which offer advice on nutrition and administer limited health services; home nursing, with needed equipment provided by local authorities; domestic help and night attendants; laundry services for the bedridden and infirm; and podiatry services. Some of these services are available in parts of the United States, but, as our study of home health services in the District of Columbia showed, they are haphazardly organized, understaffed, and inadequate.

Perhaps the most important parts of the British system of health care for the elderly are not available in this country to any significant extent. For an aged Englishman who does not need institutional care but who has regular medical needs to be met, the government has established "day hospitals," which offer physical and occupational therapy. Transportation to and from the day hospital is provided by ambulance. England also has Psychogeriatric Assessment units where a patient can be examined by both a geriatric physician and a psychiatrist, who then decide whether the patient need enter an institution (a mental hospital or nursing home) or whether, with help, he can manage in the community. Although these units are not yet universally available in the United Kingdom, they are becoming more and more common.

Nursing homes and hospitals are the last resorts. All district general hospitals have geriatric units that provide consultation and advice to outpatients, and, if necessary, admit the patient to twenty-four-hour hospital care geared to his special needs. Nursing homes are reserved for those who are totally unable to live indedendently or with help and need constant but not intensive care, or who are recuperating after a hospital stay.

Simply keeping the aged out of institutions is not enough. All these efforts, some of which are expensive, are predicated on the belief that a person does not lose his social worth simply because he is old, that the aged can make contributions to society and to themselves, and that these contributions more than pay back the costs of programs to keep them in society.

In Britain six out of ten persons over sixty-five want to continue working. Throughout the country, voluntary organizations, industries, and commercial firms have developed work schemes for the elderly. Employment exchanges have been set up to encourage the employment of older workers, and many voluntary bureaus keep records of employers willing to hire the elderly. Local government and labor unions have collaborated to establish, advise, and assist work programs that provide full-time light work for the elderly.

For those who do not wish to continue working, a preretirement association, in collaboration with some companies, offers courses for the preparation for retirement, and social and cultural activities. Adult education is arranged for the aged by local educational authorities and such organizations as the Workers Education Association. A great variety of social and luncheon clubs, day centers, and volunteer work programs help to keep the retired person active physically and socially. Free radios are distributed to the blind and bedridden through two charitable organizations. All in all, the United Kingdom has done a great deal to help retired persons use what they have most of: leisure time.

In England the special housing needs of the aged are also given an attention that in the United States is rare. About five hundred voluntary housing associations are building housing units specially equipped for aged tenants, units that have handrails near bath tubs, easy-to-open windows, low cupboards, good heating, and a bell alarm to the building warden's headquarters. The units are small and easy to care for; most have one bed/sitting room, kitchen, and bath, but those for married couples have two rooms, kitchen, and bath. In other parts of the country "boarding-out schemes," whereby private households take in elderly persons, have been established.

Britain has a pension system much like ours, with earnings-related social security benefits. The program carries an earnings limit; those who work beyond retirement age receive a smaller pension, as in this country. A supplementary pension, designed to bring a person's income to a guaranteed weekly level, is given to those who are above the minimum retirement age, not in full-time work, and cannot manage on their incomes. Certain tax relief is given to people over sixty-five of low income, and money is available to the elderly taxpayer whose daughter lives in his home and looks after him. There are, finally, many financial concessions for retired persons: rate and rent rebates, operated by housing authorities to benefit people with low incomes; transportation fare reductions (and sometimes free transportation); reduced prices for movies, the theater, and so on. And, of course, medical costs are taken care of.

Most of the programs and opportunities for the aged in the United Kingdom are available in this country as well. Both nations have old-age pension and welfare systems; both have programs to obtain jobs for those who want to work; both are engaged in some building of low-income housing for the elderly. What is important to note is not the number of programs but their scope, and the coordination among the various programs. Partly because Great Britain has had a much longer tradition of governmental assistance to the people and partly because it is a smaller nation, an immeasurably better job is done of seeing that services reach the people they are designed to reach. In England, every district hospital has a geriatric unit; in the United States, if there is a geriatric hospital unit near an older person who needs one, it is merely coincidental. We have no national health policy to insure that services are widely and equitably distributed throughout this country, and, as a result, medical facilities, like social welfare programs, tend to cluster together. Other quirks of history and economics have made the American system less effective than the British; in this country, labor unions have been extremely interested in lowering the retirement age and increasing retirement pensions, but they have done much less to provide after-retirement activities or education for their members than their English counterparts. The long English tradition of housekeepers has helped to keep that country from the critical shortage of such assistance in America.

There is no good excuse for the intolerable neglect foisted upon elderly people in this country; if we are long on retirement and short on retirement activities, if we are short of housekeepers and home nurses, it is because our people have not wanted to supply them. In the continued absence of a coherent, thoughtful, and humane national health policy, even the most well-intentioned efforts of governments, organizations, and individuals will miss the mark as often as they hit it, and confusion and ineffectiveness will continue to be the order of the day.

DENMARK

Denmark shares with Britain a concern to help the aged to live in their own homes for as long as possible. The Care of Invalidity and Old-Age Pensioners Act of

April 15, 1964 (revised in 1968), provides that the local authorities shall:

(1) Inform a pensioner who has been awarded an invalidity or old-age pension about his rights, not only under the 1968 Act, but also under other rules relevant to pensioners;

(2) Inform a pensioner about to be admitted to an old people's home or nursing home about the rules applying to the clientele of the home;

(3) Assist the pensioner in arranging his dwelling so as to make it better suited as a home for the pensioner;

(4) Assist him in purchasing any necessary health aids, such as bandages, supporting corsets, and, if appropriate, a telephone;

(5) Grant home help, as required;

(6) Ensure the availability of the necessary number of places in old people's homes and nursing homes;

(7) Make payments, if necessary, toward special expenses for help to invalids and pensioners living in blocks of service flats especially intended for that category of the population;

(8) Provide or support welfare services for disabled and elderly persons;

(9) Pay, in whole or in part, seasons tickets for public means of transport for pensioners in their areas.

Like the English, the Danes have a Home Health Service, which provides home nursing, chiropodists, and general practitioners to cure minor infirmities before they become serious. A number of other services supply housekeeping care independent of medical services.

In most of the nation's large cities, education courses are offered to the aged for a minimal charge. The Social Welfare Administration conducts two-week programs called "Folk Highschool Attendance," in which older people study current affairs. An independent Danish organization purchases unsold airline tickets and resells them to the aged at a considerable reduction. Local authorities are also empowered to provide or support activities for retired persons, such as meetings and lectures, films, club activities, social gatherings, excursions, physical exercise, home visits, and so forth. These activities are generally free of charge.

Although Denmark has constructed a number of pensioner flats, the number is still inadequate to meet the demand, and one must apply through the welfare office and prove financial need in order to be eligible. Under the Rent Subsidy Act, tenants are granted financial help if their rent exceeds a specific proportion of their income; not all housing is covered by this act, but interest-free loans and rent allowances are available to tenants in other housing. The Danes have also constructed service flats, in which each resident has his own apartment in a building with a common restaurant and free meal delivery. The full possibilities of this kind of miniature community have only begun to be explored in Denmark, although they are far advanced in Sweden. The most exciting Danish experiment involves integrating nursing home units with the service flats, so that the transition from the independence of an apartment into nursing home care and vice versa is gradual and gentle, and—even more important—so that admission to a nursing home no longer means that an elderly person loses all contact with the place, the people, and the society he knows.

Perhaps the most important contribution of Denmark to the care of the aged is also the simplest, and could easily be attempted in the United States. In Denmark, public health and welfare officers regularly inspect not only nursing homes but also the conditions of the patients; inspections are unannounced.

SWEDEN

Although Sweden, like Denmark and the United Kingdom, helps its aged avoid institutionalization through home care services, the nation's unique contribution derives from the structure of the institutions it has created. Home health care for the elderly in Sweden consists of three basic services: occupational therapy; basic medical care, such as injections, changing of bandages, and so on; and help with personal hygiene from home helpers under the supervision of registered nurses.

These services, which used to be offered by three different administrations, have recently been combined to prevent fragmentation of services. The United States could try such consolidated services, at least on a regional basis.

Compared to the home health services offered in Great Britain, those in Sweden are not so complete; they are complemented, however, by excellent institutional care. The nursing homes are of high caliber and increasingly are being designed so as to blur the line between institutionalization and independence. New centers for the aged have been built with apartments surrounding a central service unit that provides facilities for medical care, hobbies, therapy, baths, hairdressing, gymnastics, and even banking. Dependent residents live in single rooms plus bath or in complete apartments if only partially dependent. Community activities are encouraged through sales of articles made by residents and through the facilities of the service unit—library, music room, films, television, billiards, cafeteria, restaurant, pub, and auditorium. Four major industries in Malmö, the southernmost of Sweden's three major cities, built such a collective center for their pensioned employees. Its two residential buildings are joined by a third that houses porters, cleaners, a restaurant, and a full-time nurse. A doctor is available at all times at standard rates. Guest rooms, studies, billiards, television, and a library are provided. Residents are eligible for home improvement loans; the welfare administration provides grants for home remodeling and social workers to handicapped persons.

In Malmö, too, a new kind of nursing home is being developed and tested by the government. The city is building a three-million-dollar "old peoples' center" to replace the nursing home. The theory behind the project is that institutionalized old people do not need more regulation than others. The center's restaurant, for example, has applied for a liquor license—a revolutionary step. The center is designed to resemble a hotel. Its operation has been taken from the social welfare administration and put into the hands of the Medical Service Board, which provides various consultant specialists.

Although the center is having problems completing its staff, it is well under way.

All these remarkable attempts to change the nature of the nursing home fundamentally are complemented by another program that could be easily worked into the present structure of nursing home care in America. In an effort to keep patients active, involved in their society, and in control of some parts of their environment, Swedish nursing homes sponsor "Joint Councils" —meetings where patients can discuss their situation with the management of their home or with representatives of the government, making complaints, offering suggestions, and participating generally in the operation of the home. (The Danes have adopted a similar program, in which residents are permitted to discuss their homes directly with local authorities, without consulting the administrator of the home. The situation in both countries is immeasurably better than that in this country, where complaint procedures are so fragmented and bureaucratized as to be practically useless.)

Offered, too, are the usual activities programs: handicrafts, sports, dramatics, adult education, and so on. Ready-cooked meals are distributed to paid subscribers in parts of the country. In urban areas such as Malmö, door-to-door transportation services can be obtained.

Sweden has an old-age pension, which is computed from a base sum that follows the general level of prices and is revised monthly to reflect changes in the cost of living. A similar program has often been advocated but never passed in the United States. Sweden pays an old-age disability allowance or an advanced pension for an injured or blind person who is incapable of looking after himself and needs regular help. An allowance given by local authorities provides assistance in meeting costs of housing, nursing home care, and supervision of sick persons in institutions. Retired persons are also entitled to sick benefits, and, with certain restrictions, reduced fare on railways and some boats, buses, and trams.

In none of these countries is life ideal after sixty-five; we have tried to emphasize, however, the diversity of approaches in the three nations, and suggest specific programs that seem especially relevant to American problems. It is well to remember that although a creative, flexible program can immeasurably improve life for the aged, no program, however imaginative and well-supported, can solve all problems. In both England and Sweden, as in the United States, contact between the young and the old is deteriorating; traditional family patterns are breaking down; urbanization has left rural areas of Sweden with many old people and few young; suburbanization has left the central cities to the aged while the young go to the suburbs. These problems are as familiar to Americans as they are to Englishmen, Danes, and Swedes; and it is difficult to imagine a social welfare program that could meet the difficulties of a society segregated by age. The English and Swedes, at least, are experimenting. In both nations, housing for the elderly is increasingly being built in juxtaposition with housing occupied by the young, while in the United States institutional and community segregation continues to grow. It is too early to assess the effects of these European experiments, but it is not too early to start some experiments of our own.

5 Recommendations and Conclusions

The government, the nursing home industry, and the medical profession must make deliberate and concerted efforts to make nursing homes truly "homes" for the elderly, and not just places where older Americans wait to die.

We recommend strict Federal enforcement of present standards for nursing homes receiving Federal funds; this would mean elimination of the "substantial compliance" approval given homes that are in violation of the law. We recognize that cutting off funds to substandard nursing homes may in the short run leave some Medicare and Medicaid patients with no alternatives, but the route of expediency taken by the Federal government has failed spectacularly to achieve the goal of upgrading these institutions. Stricter measures are in order, with contingency plans for caring for patients after cessation of payments to violators. The necessary expenditure for placing displaced patients in hospitals or specially licensed private homes will be more than compensated for if nursing homes are forced in the long run to offer acceptable levels of care. Given vigorous leadership by Federal authorities, and eliminating discretionary clauses, local and state inspectors may often be able to gain improvements without resorting to cutting off funds. Training of inspectors, as proposed by the Public Health

Service, should be encouraged and vastly expanded as a means of making standards uniform throughout the country.

As another incentive to homes to achieve high-quality care, the Department of Health, Education and Welfare (HEW) should publish ratings for homes that receive Federal funds. Quality ratings, along with a label of the level of care offered, would also help the elderly avoid an unfortunate choice through ignorance.

Medical review should be implemented by HEW, and the medical profession should cooperate in making such a review a viable and efficient exercise of professional responsibility to insure adequate policies and practices in nursing homes.

Training of aides is another area where much remains to be done. The crucial role of the aide makes in-service education a priority item in any campaign for improving nursing homes. Medicare presently requires that aides be trained, but as both our research and our experiences showed us, training is usually haphazard and often non-existent.

As licensing of administrators gets under way, state governments have the responsibility for seeing that high standards are set, especially for educational qualifications. The nursing home industry should use the licensing process as a means of attracting qualified administrators. It should also support educational programs for health administrators. To meet the goals envisioned by the licensing law, the Federal government should tighten its regulations to insure that no single interest group dominates the state licensing boards.

Congress and HEW should also consider a better means of identifying owners of nursing homes, and of holding them legally accountable for conditions in their homes. Entrance contracts by which a patient irrevocably signs away his property should be clarified through legal means.

The Food and Drug Administration should exercise strict control over experimental drug research on nursing home patients. The FDA should require more rigid proof of consent from responsible persons and full, direct involvement of physicians who, along with the homes, should be held accountable for the effects of drug experiments on patients.

Finally, the Federal government should actively promote alternatives for the elderly outside the nursing home—"integrated" community housing through Model Cities and other programs, employment opportunities, home care programs, for example. At the present time, Congress has not allotted the elderly their fair share of these public services.

There is no question that we must invest more resources in improving the lot of the elderly. But this cost need not be an overwhelming burden. Millions of dollars are now wasted by a chaotic government apparatus that administers programs, particularly health services, dealing with the elderly. A clear national health policy and centralization of programs for the elderly could eliminate waste as well as provide better public services.

Expenditures to enforce standards in nursing homes would help insure that the massive Federal support of these institutions is actually buying good care, not merely enriching the coffers of private industry. Enforced standards would also help eliminate abuses— higher charges for government-subsidized patients or outsize drug charges, for example.

Although a new emphasis on preventive medicine and rehabilitative care would be costly in the short run, it would be partially offset by reducing the high cost of caring for persons who become incapacitated and critically ill. More psychiatric treatment for the elderly, for example, could reduce personnel problems in nursing homes as well as many medical costs for disturbed older patients by increasing the efficiency with which care is delivered. Administrators of Medicare and Medicaid are already finding that strict enforcement measures, including medical review, are well worth the investment in terms of better and more efficient care.

Outside the institution, service programs involving the elderly would add rich new resources to communities. A budget-conscious Congress should be aware that today the elderly represent some of our most wasted human resources. A national commitment to serve the elderly could meet a serious national problem: the demoralization of becoming old. No nation can afford to throw away 10 per cent of its population, as we now tend to do.

Government reorganization to improve public health services is one of the first requirements in an effort to help the elderly. In the following pages, we have outlined recommendations that seem to us of special importance. They are important because we believe that the Federal government is going to have to answer the problems of care for the aged. The default of private interests such as the medical profession and the nursing home industry means that the effort must be a public one; the reluctance or inability of the states to lead in this matter means that the problems must be solved at the national level.

GOVERNMENT REORGANIZATION

One of the major problems confronting the aged in our society is the fact that their needs are not being voiced or taken care of by one consolidated organization. For example, there are over twenty-two bureaus and agencies within the United States Department of Health, Education and Welfare alone, which are concerned, to varying degrees, with one or more aspects of the health needs of the elderly.[1] The result is a great fragmentation of responsibility; communication between bureaus and departments is a major problem. Few employees are aware of what other bureaus are doing, what information they have, and whether their efforts are being duplicated.

Since each bureau is limited in its responsibility, it is exceedingly difficult to acquire an overview of the entire field. It has been suggested that another bureau be established in HEW for the purpose of coordinating efforts, minimizing duplication, and channeling information to those directly responsible for a particular subject. This bureau would be made available to the public as well as to all HEW employees, for many citizens have spent unnecessary time trying to locate the best source of information for their inquiry.

On an interdepartmental level, the same lack of communication, and the same duplication of efforts occurs.

It is inevitable that some lack of communication will occur within such a large complex, but efforts must be made to improve interdepartmental communication and project coordination. The President's Task Force on Aging recommends that:

> . . . the heads of the human resources agencies—the Department of Health, Education and Welfare; Housing and Urban Development; Labor; Transportation; and Agriculture; and the Office of Economic Opportunity— develop organizational mechanisms capable of: 1) inter-relating each of the programs of their agencies which affect the elderly; 2) assuring that planning undertaken by their agencies does not neglect the elderly; and 3) call-ing the needs of the elderly to the attention of key decision-makers.[2]

To unify the health needs of the elderly under one agency, the Task Force and others have suggested that a separate Federal department of health be established for the purpose of coordinating all Federal health pro-grams under a single cabinet-level officer.

The HEW Task Force on Medicaid and Related Programs stated that a separate department would be inadvisable for three major reasons:

> 1. A separate Department of Health would be a prime target for "capture" by powerful special-interest groups. Struggles over key appointments in the health field attest to the stakes involved. As part of a larger agency, health activities are frequently subjected to close scrutiny and countervailing forces which can act as a shield against powerful interest groups. Many mayors and governors, recognizing this problem, are integrating their Health Departments into multi-functional agencies.
>
> 2. Health programs are deeply affected by activities of other HEW programs, e.g., income maintenance, edu-cation, and social welfare services. A separate health department would probably make coordination among such programs more difficult.
>
> 3. Many Federal health programs in other agencies belong where they are located—as, for example, in the Armed Forces and Veteran's Administration. Transfer of such programs might be less effective than it would be to offer the senior Federal health officer an opportunity to influence all Federal health policy. In any case, the real

influence of the Federal health chief is more likely to depend on the credibility, capability and strength of his operation than on his title.[3]

Others have suggested an undersecretary of health within HEW. The Subcommittee on Executive Reorganization and Government Research, of the Committee on Government Operations of the United States Senate, recommended:

> Reorganizing the Department of Health, Education and Welfare, to provide for an Under-Secretary for Health with four assistant Secretaries responsible for the following functions: budget and planning; science, manpower, and education; health care services; consumer protection. An Under-Secretary would bring new status to the health function of the Department and permit him to better organize the efforts of the agency with primary responsibility for this mission.[4]

The President's Task Force on the Aging is also concerned with the lack of coordination at the Federal level. The Task Force noted that

> [no agency exists with the] authority to determine priorities, to settle conflicts, to eliminate duplication, to identify and assign responsibility, to search for gaps within and between agencies, to initiate concerted action, to keep Federal agencies constantly aware of how their programs affect the elderly.
>
> The Task Force recognizes that in enacting the Older Americans Act, Congress intended the Administration on Aging to serve as the Federal focal point on aging. The experience of the Administration on Aging during the last four years, however, makes it abundantly clear that interdepartmental coordination cannot be carried out by a unit of government which is subordinate to the units it is attempting to coordinate. Nor does the experience of the President's Council on Aging suggest that such coordination can be accomplished effectively through such a committee.
>
> We, therefore, recommend that the President establish an Office on Aging within the Executive Office of the President. We recommend that the President seek statutory authority for this office through an amendment to the Older Americans Act but that until such authority can be obtained the President create the Office by issuing an Executive Order.

We recommend that the responsibilities of this Office include: 1) the development of national policy on aging; 2) the overseeing of planning and evaluation of all Federal activities related to aging; 3) the coordination of such activities; 4) the recommendation of priorities to the President; and 5) the encouragement of Federal agencies to undertake research and manpower preparation. We recommend that in addition the Office advise the President on concerns of the aging and alert other government officials to the potential impact of their decisions on the interests of older persons. In our judgment these responsibilities warrant Cabinet-level status for this Office.[5]

Many of those concerned with the aged question the fact that the House of Representatives has not created a select committee on aging, but instead has been content to scatter the problems of the aged among at least five different committees.[6] The Senate has had a Special Committee on Aging since March, 1961. Representative David Pryor has proposed the establishment of such a committee in the House. This task force recommends strongly that Congress grant Pryor top priority next session for the reintroduction of his proposal, and that swift approval follow.

Another major topic that is being discussed is the lack of a national health insurance policy in the United States. The Subcommittee on Executive Reorganization and Government Research stated on April 30, 1970, that:

There is no national health policy to provide form and direction to Federal health programs and expenditures. And that there is no central body or group within the executive branch that is responsible for developing Federal health policy and evaluating Federal performance in light of that policy.[7]

The Chairman of the Subcommittee sent a questionnaire to twenty-four departments and agencies. To the question about implementation and formulation of a national health policy, Dr. Shannon, who answered the questionnaire, said:

Up to and including the present, there has never been a formulation of national health policy, as such. In addition, no specific mechanism has been set up to carry out this function. As a consequence, the national health policy is a more or less amorphous set of health goals, which are derived by various means and groups within the Federal structure. In the absence of specific mechanisms for national health policy formulation, the role has been served over the years by the President, the Congress, and the Federal agencies with health responsibilities, acting individually or in various combinations as necessary.[8]

Dr. Shannon also stated that Federal health programs operated in a policy "void," and that central responsibility was "avoided." The absence of a central policy-making body for health, Dr. Shannon pointed out, has resulted in "an inability to determine goals, develop programs that support them, achieve a balance among research, education, and medical services, estimate the cost of these programs, and evaluate their performance. The tendency has been for slogans, rather than goals, to emerge," he said, adding that "slogans are poor substitutes." [9] These shortcomings virtually guarantee that Federal health programs have little relationship to each other, and are unresponsive to the health care needs of the population.

Health care organization and delivery are critical areas in need of major improvement, yet both HEW and the Federal government allocate them only 1 per cent of their health budgets. Thus, the apparent effect of the $18.8 billion Federal health budget for fiscal 1970 (and presumably the $20.6 billion budget for fiscal 1971) is to support patterns of health care and service that are outmoded and ineffective. In so doing, the current crisis in health care is compounded. Therefore, the Subcommittee recommended:

Establishing a high-level council within the executive branch, such as the Council of Health Advisors, that would be responsible for formulating and evaluating the performance of the Federal health bureacracy and its programs within the context of that policy. The Council should also recommend to the President actions to implement the national health policy.[10]

The HEW Task Force recommended much the same:

There is an urgent need to establish a National Council of Health Advisors responsible for assessing the Nation's health status and the status of the health system, for assisting in generating national health goals, and for outlining health-care objectives applicable generally to Federal health programs. The Council would consist of a small number of people broadly representative and highly qualified, having a public point of view, and appointed by the President. The Council should report to the Secretary of HEW and issue an annual report to the Nation.[11]

"National health insurance" is an expression that is becoming more widely discussed as the costs of the present health care programs have soared drastically since the inception of the Medicare and Medicaid programs in 1965. The HEW Task Force Report of June, 1970, suggested that the Department of Health, Education and Welfare:

. . . develop a policy position on this critical and controversial health-care issue. Such policy is necessary as a measure against which to appraise the proposals which Congress will soon be considering. It also seems necessary that the Department assume the initiative on an issue so central to its responsibilities.[12]

The HEW Task Force therefore recommended:

That the Secretary appoint a high-level body to undertake promptly a study directed towards development of a health-care financing policy for the Nation. The group should be composed of persons who can command the country's respect for their expertise, knowledge, and demonstrated competence in the subject matter assigned. It should not be selected to represent the various interests affected. The representational function is better served through other available channels. The group should be furnished an able full-time staff of technically qualified people. It should plan to complete its work and present recommendations to the Secretary in time to be ready for consideration during the 1971 session of the Congress.[13]

The President's Task Force on the Aging proposed that:

The Health Services and Mental Health Administration establish within the National Center for Health Services Research and Development a Council for the study of the organization, planning, management financing, and delivery of care for the elderly. [The Task Force also recommended] that within a reasonable period of time this

Council design, conduct, and report on large-scale experiments concerning comprehensive coverage, incentives for comprehensive care which could be added to existing health programs, and the effect of removing or reducing the deductible and co-insurance features of Medicare.[14]

The Senate Subcommittee on Executive Reorganization and Government Research also suggested:

eliminating all health-related functions of the Commerce Department's Economic Development Administration and the Small Business Administration and transferring these functions to HEW. The funds spent by EDA and SBA on health should be kept in the agency and allocated to agency functions that have been underfunded.[15]

This last recommendation would help to unify citizens' health needs under one department.

Data on long-term care are scattered through all the different agencies administering the various health programs for the elderly. The HEW Task Force stated that:

. . . the data available on long-term care resources, services and expenditures are fragmentary and generally inadequate. D/HEW supports extensive programs which provide institutional and home-based long-term care services, and very considerable private funds are involved in paying for these services also. What are these programs yielding? Are the results related to the expenditure levels? How are these services financed? Is their distribution adequate and are they accessible to persons who need them? The growing need and the increasing demand for these services and the relationship between long-term care, hospital and medical care in general, highlight the need for more usable program management information.

Three agencies of D/HEW collect some long-term care data. The Office of Research and Statistics of the Social Security Administration publishes national health expenditures data, considerable related data derived from Medicare coverage in extended care facilities and home health agencies. The National Center for Social Statistics collected program data derived from public assistance programs, which include skilled nursing home, intermediate care and homemaker services. The National Center for Health Statistics assembles data on nursing home facilities —their number, bed capacity, staff patterns and other characteristics. A number of other D/HEW components provide some management information for their own programs, as do agencies of several other Government Departments.

However, none of these agencies have the mandate to systematize the information available, or to attempt to fill some of the substantial gaps in data needed to assess program validity. The Office of Research and Statistics of the Social Security Administration is viewed as the most natural and competent resource for coordinative effort because of its close relationship with medical-care and social insurance programs and because of established research capability.[16]

Therefore, the HEW Task Force recommended that:

A major effort should be undertaken with D/HEW to systematize, coordinate and improve the collection and analysis of data dealing with nursing home and other post-hospital and long-term care resources, expenditures and services. This should include information from all relevant governmental and non-governmental sources.[17]

THE INFORMATION DELIVERY SYSTEM

Communicating information to a large group of people has always been a problem in our society. Although referral services and information centers publicize the services available to them, many elderly Americans are unaware of the benefits to which they are entitled, and they often do not understand the nature of these benefits. Therefore, many elderly are not taking full advantage of the resources available to them.

The President's Task Force on the Aging recommended an innovative approach to delivering such information to the elderly.

We recommend that in addition to other community information and referral services the Social Security Administration establish a system for delivering information through its District Offices to older persons and their families concerning the availability of benefits and services for the elderly. We recommend that the costs of the system be paid from the general revenues. We further recommend that, wherever feasible, the Social Security Administration contract for performance of this function older persons to be employed or utilized as volunteers on a priority basis.[18]

If a program such as this were implemented effectively, it would benefit not only the elderly and their families but nursing home administrators as well. An administrator in a home in Maryland said that the Social Security District Offices often mislead the children of potential nursing home patients by oversimplifying the eligibility requirements for the Medicare extended care benefits. On more than one occasion, families have called this administrator, asking that their mothers be admitted for one hundred days of Medicare services. The nursing home administrator must then explain all the details of eligibility, and the families often feel that the home is cheating them.[19] A Social Security Administration official admitted to this during an interview, but said that corrective measures were being taken in the form of detailed instruction pamphlets to the District Offices.[20]

EDUCATION OF HEALTH PROFESSIONALS

In many nursing homes we visited, either the head nurse or administrator told us that one of their major problems was staffing the facility with qualified, concerned personnel. This problem is linked to the education given each professional in the health field.

Talking to medical students and doctors who teach at medical schools, we found that geriatrics is the least popular course of study. More interested professors are needed in the field of geriatrics to attract larger numbers of medical students, who usually turn away from this field early in their studies. It should be required that a medical student do part of his training with geriatric patients so that he will at least have come in contact with this age group. The intern will then have a broader, more balanced knowledge of the medical spectrum, and will be better equipped to deal with decisions of specialization. This training requirement would also help alleviate some of the staffing shortages in nursing homes, and, if combined with a medical review team, could significantly improve the quality of care offered in nursing homes.

The Group for the Advancement of Psychiatry recommended:

> Training and education of all the health professions—nursing, social work, medicine, occupational therapy, psychiatry, psychology—must include didactic coverage of both the phenomenon of aging and the nature of the elderly. Health manpower must be increased in number as well as quality. The National Institute of Mental Health, in particular, should be provided sufficient budget and personnel to take an active catalytic role in effecting changes in education, in community health centers, and other areas. New kinds of schools for health practitioners are mandatory.[21]

There should also be retraining programs for doctors so that they can keep up with the times. And, as some states require periodic driving tests in order to renew our driving licenses, periodic license renewal for doctors should also be required by law. In addition, it might be a good idea for high schools to provide students with a health course on some basic first-aid facts. A television series of lectures devoted to home care and first aid would also be an effective means of instructing the public.

CONSUMER PROTECTION FOR THE ELDERLY

The elderly are vulnerable consumers. According to the President's Task Force on the Aging:

> Particularly vicious are attempts to sell older persons goods and services for which they have no need. Published documented reports of such exploitation include: land fraud, patent medicines, physical therapy devices, fraudulent insurance, and home remodeling. The Task Force believes that all levels of government must act more strenuously to protect the limited financial resources of older persons. One such action is to educate older persons to protect themselves.
>
> Some of the elderly have special problems in the marketplace. The Task Force finds the connection between susceptibility to fraud and loneliness and chronic illness a particularly sad commentary on the way many older Americans spend their last years. While consumer education and protection are important for all persons,

experience has shown that those who need it most, especially the elderly, are the hardest to reach.[22]

Therefore, the President's Task Force recommended "that the proposed Office of Consumer Affairs, the Department of Health, Education and Welfare, and the Office of Economic Opportunity mount an intensive campaign heavily emphasizing outreach techniques to offer consumer education and protection to the elderly."[23]

CONSUMER REPRESENTATION IN HEALTH POLICY-MAKING

The HEW Task Force has a number of recommendations concerning consumer representation. The Task Force report stated:

> When one talks of the need for policy, goals, boundaries, tradeoffs and controls, the question arises as to who makes the ultimate decisions. The answer varies with the problem, and obviously with the distinction between clinical and public policy situations. However, with more sophistication, greater access to the facts and more experience, the consumer in health, as in education wants a greater voice in matters affecting his well-being and his pocketbook. With the advent of massive public financing of health services through Congressional enactments in recent years, public decision-making in the health services became inevitable, and public decision-making without consumer participation is like an election without votes.[24]

The HEW Task Force believes that:

> . . . all consumers should have access to health care without hardship or humiliation and as far as possible with some voice in how it is planned and some choice of how it is furnished.
>
> The fact is that millions of consumers get care on a hit-or-miss basis; millions more lack access to care except in medical crises; and virtually all consumers lack access to the decision-making machinery that can bring about change.
>
> . . . The size of the gap in consumer access to the decision-making machinery of health care is apparent from the fact that few institutions and programs include users of their services on policy-making or governing

boards, in spite of their nonprofit and presumably "community" character. The result is that medical care is still too often delivered at the time and place, and in the way convenient to provider rather than to consumer. Old patterns persist in the face of new demands—a basic cause of rising dissatisfaction with the health services.[25]

. . . Health institutions and programs must learn to live with the fact that their consumers are going to have a real voice in planning and evaluating health services. While we recognize the inevitability of consumer participation and have seen examples of the valid contributions consumers have made to the effectiveness of health services, we are also aware of the misgivings of many health professionals who doubt that consumers can make substantive contributions and some who fear actual obstruction.[26]

Therefore, the HEW Task Force recommended:

Any board or group set up to advise policy-making officials at any level of Government or of health-care agencies sponsored by Government must include consumer representatives to protect and present the interests and needs of the consumer. The consumer representatives selected to serve on policy-making and advisory boards should reflect the social, economic, racial and geographic characteristics of their community.

Federal, state and non-governmental agencies involved in planning, delivering, and purchasing health services should make provision for special orientation programs for new members of policy-making groups, including the consumer representatives on such groups.

Programs of health education should be considered integral components of health-care services and all providers receiving Federal support should be required to provide continuing programs of health education to their consumers.[27]

H.R. 17550 Bill passed by the House of Representatives on May 21, 1970, and now pending in the Senate, provides for consumer representatives in a program review team.

For the purposes of paragraph (1) (B) and (C) of this subsection, and clause (F) of section 1866(b)(2), the Secretary shall, after consultation with appropriate State and local professional societies, the appropriate carriers and intermediaries utilized in the administration of this title, and consumer representatives familiar with the health needs of residents of the State, appoint one or more program review teams (composed of physicians, other professional personnel in the health care field, and consumer representatives) in each State.[28]

TRANSPORTATION NEEDS OF THE ELDERLY

The Special Committee on Aging of the United States Senate, called the transportation problem of the aged "forced immobility." [29] According to the Committee Report, these are the major transportation difficulties of the elderly:

1. Cost—which limits mobility for those on limited fixed incomes. This related to employment for those who need a little extra work to supplement Social Security payments, participation in education, recreation and social events, visiting family, friends, clinics, physicians, hospitals, shopping, etc. We have proposed reduced fares during the non-rush hours which we believe would create greater movement and increase business as well as relieve some of the isolation existing among older people. Even with permissive legislation now in existence, we have been unsuccessful in our efforts to reduce cost.

2. Schedules—during weekdays and Sundays long waits are necessary involving time and exposure especially dangerous to health in bad weather.

Many people are deprived of work and opportunity to worship in their own churches because they have no way to get there.

3. Routing—involving two fares are an extra drain on the pocketbook and limit older people to their own living areas or neighborhood.

4. Lack of safety in the loading and unloading zones is often reported. Many complain of the difficulty of getting on and off buses. The handicapped are virtually isolated because of this problem.[30]

Some of the obvious travel barriers are the high steps on buses, fast-moving subway escalators, unsheltered bus stops, lurching vehicles, and so on. Some suggestions have been made for improvements in the public transportation system to benefit the elderly and the physically handicapped, who now number more than six million. Among suggested improvements were sheltered benches, subway gates, no-step buses, well-spaced poles in the buses, computerized speeds controlling gradual acceleration and deceleration, and one-way doors.[31]

The Senate Report recommended that:

[since] Transportation problems among older Americans have reached the critical stage in many metropolitan and rural regions of the United States, Federal agencies have made a beginning in identifying problems, initiating research, and conducting pilot programs to test systems and concepts. The overall problem, however, is so serious that the following additional actions should be taken:

Technical assistance should be provided by appropriate Federal agencies to acquaint municipal governing bodies and private transportation managers with facts about transit barriers, special needs of the elderly and the handicapped, and new transportation concepts which would benefit, not only the elderly, but all persons who use public transportation.

The Urban Mass Transit Administration should submit to the Congress its recommendations for removing travel barriers and using existing and potential mass transit legislation to promote worthwhile social purposes . . .

Provision should be made in planning the 1971 White House Conference on Aging for a preliminary report on transportation, to be prepared by a panel capable of giving adequate attention to sociological, technical, and psychological aspects of the subject. Every attempt should be made to show the relationship of transportation to service programs, existing or contemplated, for older Americans.[32]

The Senate Report also recommended that:

The U.S. Department of Transportation, in conjunction with the Department of Health, Education and Welfare, its Administration on Aging, and the Department of Housing and Urban Development, seek ways of providing necessary transportation for the elderly and other disadvantaged groups who are not within reach of, or able to use normal public transportation (if it exists) in order to take advantage of nutrition, health and other services.[33]

In its legislative objectives for 1970, the American Association of Retired Persons stated: "We urge that all Federal, state and local agencies give special attention to the needs of older persons with respect to the cost, availability, suitability, and proximity of public transportation." [34] The President's Task Force on Aging recommendation was similar to the recommendations made by the Senate:

> We recommend that the President direct the Departments of Transportation, Housing and Urban Development, and Health, Education and Welfare, and the Office of Economic Opportunity to undertake jointly an intensive time-limited study of all aspects of transportation as it affects the lives of the elderly. The study should include the design and construction or modification of necessary equipment, experiments, and demonstrations. We further recommend that this study culminate in the formulation of recommendations on how best to meet the transportation needs of the elderly, so that appropriate action can be undertaken at an early date, including the submission of a program to the Congress.[35]

NATIONAL HEALTH INSURANCE

As the cost to the Federal government of providing care under the Medicare and Medicaid programs increases steadily, people have been looking for alternative methods of caring for the health of the nation. One of the alternatives proposed is national health insurance.

The Group for the Advancement of Psychiatry proposed a "Universal Prepaid Comprehensive Health Insurance." [36]

The Special Senate Committee on Aging commented:

> The Advisory Committee on Health Aspects of the Economics of Aging emphatically expressed the belief that a comprehensive, compulsory health insurance program for all age groups—a program with built-in cost controls, standards for quality care, incentives for prepaid group practice, and other badly needed reforms—"offers the best hope that this Nation has for living up to the oft expressed declaration that good health care is the right of every man, woman and child who lives in this land."
>
> But, before such a program can be established, "public and private efforts should immediately be made to deal with demonstrated deficiencies in Medicare." [37]

These reasons were given:

> 1.   Health-care problems of the elderly are still widespread and they remain urgent.

2. Three years of experience under Medicare have provided invaluable lessons in the operation of a major public health insurance program. The time has come to heed those lessons.

3. Current investigations into profiteering under Medicaid and Medicare have helped focus attention upon the need for cost controls and establishment of uniform standards of care. Such reforms can have a beneficial effect upon the entire health industry and can combat medical cost inflation.

4. Success in improving Medicare will lead to more general acceptance of steps necessary to provide higher quality health care to our entire population.

5. The lack of sufficient consumer representation in Medicare and its almost total absence from State advisory committees for Medicaid is deplorable.

National discussion about the need for a national health insurance program can serve a vital function if it turns public, professional and governmental attention to actions that must be taken to remedy deficiencies which have become more apparent as more and more Federal funds have been committed to health care.

The people of this Nation now have an opportunity to transform public concern into positive action and reform. Corrective action should begin with Medicare and Medicaid and it should aim at long-range improvements rather than hasty retrenchment.[38]

The reports and recommendations in this chapter are based on detailed studies by qualified health experts and government officials. Our own recommendations are also based on evidence gathered by commissions and task forces that have studied nursing homes. The facts are before us; what we need now is the will and determination to act. The needs of the elderly cannot wait while America appoints task forces and special commissions. Our report indicates that it is not necessary to wait; indeed, it is imperative to act now if our elderly citizens are to share fully in a national abundance they helped create.

NOTES

CHAPTER 1.

1. From 70 to 75 per cent of all extended care facilities do not meet Medicare standards, according to the Social Security Administration. Medicaid homes are reportedly even more frequently in violation of standards, although the Medical Services Administration does not compile figures on nursing home violations under Title XIX.
2. Statistics on the economics of the elderly are taken from *Developments in Aging, 1969: A Report of the Special Committee on Aging,* U.S. Senate, May 15, 1970, pp. 1–31.
3. From a speech to the U.S. House of Representatives, August 3, 1970.

CHAPTER 2.

Legislative History of National Health Insurance

1. U.S. Bureau of the Census, *Statistical Abstract of the United States: 1963* (Eighty-fourth edition, Washington, D.C., 1963).
2. Richard Harris, *A Sacred Trust* (The New American Library, New York, 1966), p. 72.
3. *Ibid.,* p. 74.
4. Peter A. Corning, *The Evolution of Medicare . . . from idea to law* (United States Government Printing Office, Washington, D.C., 1969), p. 22.
5. *Op. cit.,* Harris, p. 123.

6. *Ibid.,* p. 144.
7. *Ibid.,* p. 156.
8. *Ibid.,* p. 174.
9. *Ibid.,* p. 180.
10. *Ibid.,* p. 196.

Medicare, Medicaid, and the Nursing Home

1. Interview, Claire Townsend with Frank Frantz, Deputy Commissioner of Health, Education and Welfare Medical Services Administration, August 26, 1970.
2. There are still only about six hundred hospital-based Extended Care Facilities, according to the Bureau of Health Insurance, the Social Security Administration. Progressive care has not caught on in hospitals.
3. Interview, Claire Townsend with Val Halamanderis, staff director of the Senate Subcommittee on Long-Term Care, June 25, 1970.
4. Interview, Claire Townsend with Frank Frantz, August 26, 1970.
5. Interview, Claire Townsend with Frank Frantz, August 26, 1970.
6. *Medicare and Medicaid: Problems, Issues and Alternatives,* Report of the Staff to the Committee on Finance, U.S. Senate, February 9, 1970, p. 92.
7. *Ibid.,* pp. 92–93.
8. *Ibid.,* p. 93.
9. First Annual Report on Medicare, prepared by the Secretary of HEW, pp. 34–35.
10. Letter from Arthur E. Hess, Director of the Bureau of Health Insurance, SSA, to state agencies, December 16, 1966.
11. *Medicare and Medicaid,* p. 94.
12. Federal Regulations: Title 20, Chapter II, Part 405.1134.
13. *Ibid.,* 504.1124.
14. *Medicare and Medicaid,* p. 95.
15. *Ibid.*
16. *Ibid.*
17. Wayne Callaham, Bureau of Health Insurance, SSA, September 21, 1970.
18. Statistics compiled by the SSA, December, 1969.
19. Federal Regulations: 405.1107.
20. Interview, Claire Townsend with Mamie Dailey, Medicare inspector, Maryland, July 31, 1970.
21. Speech by Congressman David Pryor to the U.S. House of Representatives, August 3, 1970.
22. Interview, Claire Townsend with Frank Frantz, August 26, 1970.

23. Letter from Raymond Whitener, HEW employee in Illinois, to Congressman David Pryor.
24. Interview, Claire Townsend with Herbert Colton, President of Manor Care, Inc., a new nursing home chain, August 21, 1970.
25. Mal Schechter, "Default on Nursing Home Code," *Hospital Practice,* December, 1969, p. 21, column 2.
26. Report of the Staff to the Committee on Finance, *Medicare and Medicaid,* p. 42.

CHAPTER 3.

Fire in Ohio

1. Information concerning the details of the Harmar House fire was published in *Hospital Practice,* March, 1970, pp. 22–25, 30, and was made public information during hearings held in February, 1970, by the U.S. Senate Subcommittee on Long-Term Care.
2. "Fire Disaster in Ohio Home: How Good are Safety Codes?" *Hospital Practice,* March, 1970, p. 22.
3. *Ibid.,* pp. 22–23.
4. *Ibid.,* p. 30.
5. *Ibid.,* p. 22.
6. *Ibid.,* p. 23.
7. *Ibid.,* pp. 24–25.
8. Mal Schechter, *op. cit.*
9. Mr. Jack Bono, Managing Engineer for the Fire Protection Department of Underwriters' Laboratories, Inc., testifying before the Subcommittee on Long-Term Care, February 9, 1970. His testimony on the tests is as follows:

   The sample materials from [Harmar House] were subjected to three tests, the methenamine pill test, the Steiner tunnel test, and a chamber test recently developed by U.L., Inc. . . . [The first] essentially consists of exposing a 9″ x 9″ sample of the carpet to a burning methenamine pill placed in the center of the sample. Observations are made of the maximum char radius. . . . [If] Flaming did not propagate over the nylon carpeting materials tested . . . the materials would be classified as "resistant to flammability."

   The Steiner tunnel test is a national standard used for the measurement of flame spread and smoke developed of interior finish materials. It essentially consists of a rectangular furnace in which the test sample is mounted on the lid of the furnace and exposed to an igniting fire from the underside. As the test material begins to contribute to the igniting fire, flame spreads down the sample. . . . This equipment is also used to measure smoke generation during a test. A numerical limitation of 75 for the flame spread rating (based on a scale in which a non-combustible material has a zero rating and red oak flooring has a 100 rating) has been specified by the Public Health Service for regulating floor covering in hospitals receiving aid under the Hill-Burton Act . . . this test demonstrated that a sample with a backing resulted in a flame spread of 275.

The chamber test was recently developed by Underwriters' Laboratories under a research project sponsored by the Department of Health, Education and Welfare. This test exposes a sample of floor covering 2′ x 8′ in size to an impinging fire at one end. The sample is mounted in the normal floor position. Observations are made of the flame spread over the surface. . . . The degree of involvement of the carpet samples during the normal 12 minute exposure to the igniting flame was moderate. . . . However, the burning persisted after the igniting fire was shut off, and in two of three samples, the flame spread the full length of the sample. . . .

I think it can be concluded from the work of the laboratories that the nylon carpet material used in the nursing home was of a type which would not readily spread fire when exposed to a small ignition energy source such as a lighted cigarette. However, when the intensity of the heat exposure is sufficient, the nylon carpeting is capable of propagating flame.

10. According to Morris Levy, Chief of Bureau of Health Insurance, Division of State Operations; Kenneth Koppenhoeffer, Division of State Operations; James Cunningham, Community Health Service of the Public Health Service.

11. Memorandum, Dr. Joseph English, Community Health Service, PHS, to Robert Ball, Commissioner of Social Security Administration, May 6, 1970.

12. Memorandum, Dr. Harold Graning, Assistant Surgeon General, Director, Health Facilities Planning and Construction Service, PHS, to Robert Ball, Commissioner of SSA, July 9, 1970.

13. *Ibid.*

14. George Paules, President of the Carpet and Rug Institute, reprinted statement of his presentation before the

Subcommittee on the Consumer, U.S. Senate Commerce Committee, June 11, 1970.

15. George Paules, Information Council on Fabric Flammability, New York City, December 3, 1970.
16. "Moss Urges Tighter Fire Regulations for Nursing Homes," *Modern Nursing Home,* March, 1970, p. 52.
17. Memorandum, Dr. Joseph English, May 6, 1970.
18. Victor Gentilini, Public Relations Officer, National Bureau of Standards, Department of Commerce.
19. Howard Heffron, *et al., Federal Consumer Safety Legislation,* A Special Report Prepared for the National Commission on Product Safety, June, 1970, p. 147.
20. Telephone interview, Andrea Hricko with Mr. Kopelman, BHI, Division of State Operations, September 30, 1970.
21. *Ibid.*
22. Interview, Andrea Hricko with Morris Levy, September 25, 1970.

Death in Maryland

1. *Washington Post,* August 26, 1970.
2. Facts concerning the epidemic at the Gould Convalesarium are taken from *Washington Post* reports by Richard Cohen, September 18 and 19, 1970, covering hearings by the investigating panel appointed by the Maryland Department of Health and Mental Hygiene.
3. Janet Keyes attended and reported on the hearings held by the Subcommittee on Long-term Care of the Senate Committee on Aging, August 19, 1970.
4. *Ibid.*
5. *Post,* September 19, 1970, B-1.
6. *Ibid.*
7. *Post,* September 18, 1970, C-1.
8. *Ibid.*
9. *Ibid.*
10. *Ibid.*
11. *Ibid.*
12. *Ibid.*
13. Dr. Matthew Tayback, Maryland Department of Health and Hygiene, September 28, 1970.
14. Robert S. McCleery, M.D., *et al., One Life—One Physician: An Inquiry into the Medical Profession's Performance in Self-Regulation,* A Report to the Center for Study of Responsive Law (Washington, D.C., 1970), pp. 16–18.
15. Interview, Claire Townsend with Frank Frantz, Deputy

Commissioner of Medical Services Administration, August 7, 1970.
16. *Journal of Home Economics,* November, 1964, p. 653.
17. Senate hearings on Nutrition and the Aged, September 9, 1969, p. 5284.

The Administrator

1. From an advertisement for *Medical World News,* a McGraw-Hill magazine, in *Advertising Age,* July 13, 1970.
2. Brian D. Sullivan and Robert K. Byron, *Progress Report on Nursing Home Administrator Licensing Under Section 1908 of the Social Security Act* (Thesis for Yale Law School, March 15, 1970), p. 2-4.
3. *Ibid.,* p. 3-3.
4. *Ibid.,* p. 8-8.
5. *Ibid.,* p. 4-4.
6. *Ibid.,* p. 3-5.
7. *Ibid.,* p. 4-2.
8. Interview, Claire Townsend with Frank Frantz, Deputy Commissioner of Medical Services Administration, August 7, 1970.
9. Sullivan and Byron, p. 4-3.
10. *Ibid.*
11. *Ibid.,* p. 6-1.
12. *Ibid.,* p. 6-2.
13. *Ibid.,* p. 6-7.
14. *Ibid.,* p. 6-3.
15. *Ibid.,* p. 7-1.
16. *Ibid.*
17. Theodore Schuchat, "Joys and Jolts of Retirement," North American Newspaper Alliance; column for publication on August 8–9, 1970.
18. *Ibid.*
19. *Ibid.*
20. *Ibid.*
21. Interview, Claire Townsend.
22. Schuchat, *op. cit.*
23. Sid Leigh, Member of the staff of the National Advisory Council on Nursing Home Administration.
24. *Ibid.*
25. *Ibid.*

The Owners

1. 83rd Annual Report of the Presbyterian Home for Aged

Couples and Aged Persons of the State of Pennsylvania, 1967, p. 64.
2. Theodore Schuchat, "Joys and Jolts of Retirement," North American Newspaper Alliance, July 18, 1970.
3. *Ibid.*
4. J. Richard Elliott, Jr., "Unhealthy Growth?: The Nursing Home Business Is Expanding at a Feverish Pace," *Barron's,* February 10, 1969, p. 3.
5. *Ibid.*
6. J. Richard Elliott, Jr., "Wards of the State?: Healthy Growth in Nursing Homes Calls for Intensive Care," *Barron's,* March 17, 1969, p. 29.
7. J. Richard Elliott, Jr., "No Tired Blood," *Barron's,* February 24, 1969, p. 21.
8. *Ibid.,* p. 26.
9. *Ibid.*
10. *Ibid.,* p. 31.
11. *Ibid.*
12. *Ibid.,* p. 25.
13. *Ibid.,* p. 26.
14. *Ibid.,* p. 31.
15. *Ibid.*

The Personnel

1. Claire Townsend's journal.
2. *Nursing Home Fact Book* (American Nursing Home Association, 1968), p. 10.
3. Letter to Congressman David Pryor.
4. Barbara A. Davis, R.N., "Coming of Age: A Challenge for Geriatric Nursing," *Journal of the American Geriatrics Society,* 1968, pp. 1100–1106, gives an account of the rise of geriatric nursing.
5. Janet Keyes' journal.
6. Report of Subcommittee on Long-term Care, Special Committee on Aging, U.S. Senate, March, 1967, p. 43.
7. *Medicare and Medicaid: Problems, Issues and Alternatives,* Report of the Staff to the Committee on Finance, U.S. Senate, February 9, 1970, p. 67.
8. Letter to Congressman David Pryor.
9. Dr. Matthew Tayback, Maryland Department of Health and Hygiene, September 28, 1970.
10. *Ibid.*

Drugs

1. Interview, summer, 1970.
2. *Continuing Problems in Providing Nursing Home Care*

and Prescribed Drugs Under the Medicaid Program in California, 1970 General Accounting Office Audit, p. 19.

3. *Ibid.,* p. 20.

4. Report to the Subcommittee on Health of the Elderly, Special Committee on Aging (Examination into Alleged Improper Practices in Providing Nursing Home Care and Controlling Payments for Prescribed Drugs for Welfare Recipients in the State of California), U.S. Senate, August, 1966, p. 20.

5. *Ibid.*

6. *Continuing Problems,* p. 1.

7. R. M. Viola, M. F. Stein, Jr., B. Mehl, and L. S. Libow, "The Extended Care Facility (ECF) in a Teaching Public Hospital: Comparison with a Private ECF in the Same City," presented at the International Gerontological Association Meeting in Washington, D.C., August 29, 1969.

8. Interview, Margaret Quinn with Mrs. Virginia Maxwell, nursing home inspector, Montgomery County, Maryland, July 28, 1970.

9. Letter to Margaret Quinn from Mrs. Virginia Westbrook, R.N., Missouri Department of Public Health and Welfare, August 18, 1970.

10. Interview, task force members with Jim Polk, Associated Press writer, July 27, 1970.

11. Medicare regulations require that a physician visit a patient every thirty days, yet there is evidence that many visit much more infrequently. Some physicians indicate that they are depressed by conditions in nursing homes or by the old in general, and many are too busy to visit as often as needed.

12. *The Congressional Record,* March 16, 1970, E2020, which reprinted the March 8, 1970, Detroit *News* article by James Treloar.

13. *U.S. News and World Report,* July 20, 1970, p. 38.

14. *Congressional Record, loc. cit.*

15. Report to the Subcommittee on Health of the Elderly, p. 24.

16. *Continuing Problems.*

17. Interview with Jim Polk.

18. Report to the Subcommittee on Health of the Elderly, pp. 23–24.

19. Dr. George Pennebaker, California Department of Health Care Services.

20. Hearing of the Subcommittee on Medicare and Medicaid of the Senate Finance Committee, June 16, 1970.

21. Jordan Braverman, *Nursing Home Standards: A Tragic Dilemma in American Health,* American Pharmaceutical Association, Washington, D.C., 1970, pp. 50–51.
22. Medicare Regulations, Federal Register.
23. *Op. cit.,* hearing on Medicare and Medicaid.
24. Interview, Margaret Quinn with Dr. William S. Apple, Executive Director of the American Pharmaceutical Association.
25. Telephone conversation, Margaret Quinn with a Virginia pharmacist.
26. According to information received by the American Pharmaceutical Association.
27. *Op. cit.,* hearing on Medicare and Medicaid, Dr. Apple.
28. Melvin O. Moehle, "Pharmacy Discounts: Illegal? Unethical? Dishonest?" *Modern Nursing Home,* June, 1970, p. 12.
29. Letter from Dr. Apple to Clinton P. Anderson, Chairman, Subcommittee on Medicare and Medicaid, June 30, 1970; reprinted in *The APHA Newsletter,* July 11, 1970.
30. Moehle, *op. cit.*
31. Don L. McLeod, instructor in clinical pharmacy, director of the clinical and institutional extension program, School of Pharmacy, University of North Carolina.
32. Joseph A. Pollak, D. H. Lee's Rx Pharmacy, Paulding, Ohio.
33. *Op. cit.,* hearing on Medicare and Medicaid.
34. *Ibid.*
35. *Ibid.*

The Incentive to Live

1. Mother Bernadette, administrator of Saint Joseph's Manor, Trumbull, Connecticut, at a Senate hearing; reported in *The Congressional Record,* October 21, 1969.
2. Letter to Congressman David Pryor.
3. Letter to *New York Times* editor, July 10, 1970.
4. Janet Keyes' journal.
5. Interview, Janet Keyes with Dr. Robert Butler, Washington, D.C., psychiatrist and gerontologist, July 7, 1970.
6. "The Façade of Chronological Age: An Interpretative Summary," *American Journal of Psychiatry,* Vol. 119, No. 8, February, 1963, pp. 721–728.
7. "Psychiatric Contact with the Community-Resident,

Emotionally-disturbed Elderly," *Journal of Nervous and Mental Disorders,* Vol. 137, 1963, pp. 180–186.

8. Janet Keyes' journal.

9. Interview, Janet Keyes with Mrs. Monna Kohn, Administrative Assistant, Health Facilities Association of Maryland, Inc., August 20, 1970.

10. Telephone interview, Claire Townsend with Jeff Campbell, Executive Director of the West Virginia Nursing Home Association, August 8, 1970.

11. St. Joseph's Manor offers four levels of care. Its base rate for skilled nursing care is $16.00 per day or $501.00 per month; for intermediate nursing care, $9.90 per day or $301.13 a month; for Extended Care Facilities, $20.00 per day; and for hospital care, $25.00 a day. These are the rates set by the State of Connecticut for homes rated A-1. Over one-third of the patients at St. Joseph's are receiving Medicaid payments.

12. According to Arthur Barker, Deputy Chief, Facilities Survey Improvement Program, U.S. Public Health Service, September 22, 1970.

13. "Conditions of Participation; Extended Care Facilities," Federal Health Insurance for the Aged, Code of Federal Regulations, Title XX, Chapter III, Part 405; U.S. Department of Health, Education and Welfare, Social Security Administration, 405.1130 (b).

14. *Ibid.,* 405.1130(b)(3).

15. Interview, Janet Keyes with Dr. Robert Butler.

16. Letter to Claire Townsend from a nurse in an Iowa nursing home, August 19, 1970.

CHAPTER 4.

Problems of America's Aged

1. *Drug Topics,* September 28, 1970.

2. See Appendix II.

3. *Developments in Aging: 1969,* A Report of the Special Committee on Aging, U.S. Senate, February 16, 1970 (Res. 316) May 15, 1970.

4. Herman Brotman, Department of Statistics, Administration on Aging, Department of Health, Education and Welfare.

5. John B. Martin, Commissioner of the Administration on Aging, in *Aging,* 182:10, December, 1969.

6. Dr. Robert N. Butler, *Toward a Practical Ecumenism: The Older Person and His Environment: Defining the*

Goals of Service to the Aging (keynote address, Forum Session on Services to the Aging, Annual Protestant Health Association, Washington, D.C., March 3, 1970), reprinted in the *Bulletin of the American Hospital Association,* 34:6–12, 1970; and *Hospital Progress: A Journal of the Catholic Hospital Association,* July, 1970.

7. Butler, *Age-ism: Another Form of Bigotry.*
8. Interview, Elizabeth Baldwin with Pat Gilroy, Executive Director, Washington, D.C., Homemaker Service, August 10, 1970.
9. *Aging,* 182:16, December, 1969.
10. Butler, *Toward a Practical Ecumenism.*
11. A. I. Goldfarb, "Prevalence of psychiatric disorders in metropolitan old age and nursing homes," *Journal of American Geriatrics Society,* 10:77–84, 1962.
12. *Op. cit.,* Butler, *Toward a Practical Ecumenism.*
13. Beverly Bradford, "Cushioning Retirement Transition," *The Washington Post,* July 9, 1970.
14. *Ibid.*
15. Herman Brotman, *The Older Population: Some Facts We Should Know.*
16. Interview, Elizabeth Baldwin with Blue Carstonson, Executive Director of the Green Thumb Program, National Farmers Union, July 31, 1970.
17. "Hotel Evictions Continue as FIND Helps the Elderly," *Chelsea Clinton News,* April 25, 1968.
18. "Elderly Rally to FIND Program," *Chelsea Clinton News,* September 5, 1968.
19. *Ibid.*
20. *The New York Times,* May 18, 1970.

Solutions in Other Countries

1. Information in this section was obtained from *Care of the Elderly in Britain,* Reference Division, Central Office of Information, London, August, 1969; *Care of the Old and Sick,* Ministries of Labor and Social Affairs, Denmark; and *New Lives for the Old,* Yngve Tidman, Correspondent for Swedish Newspapers, Tullia Von Sydow, first Secretary of Swedish Board of Health and Welfare, Svan Thiberg, Director of Research.

CHAPTER 5.

1. See diagram of Bureaucratic Fragmentation, Appendix V.
2. *Toward a Brighter Future for the Elderly,* Report of the

President's Task Force on the Aging, April, 1970, p. 4.

3. *Recommendations of the Task Force on Medicaid and Related Programs,* United States Department of Health, Education and Welfare, June, 1970, p. 95.

4. *Federal Role In Health,* Report of the Subcommittee on Reorganization and Government Research, of the Committee on Government Operations of the United States Senate, April 30, 1970, p. 32.

5. *Op. cit.,* President's Task Force, pp. 12–13.

6. See diagram, Appendix V.

7. Reorganization Committee, *op. cit.*

8. HEW Medicaid Recommendations, *op. cit.*

9. Reorganization Committee, *op. cit.*

10. *Op. cit.,* Reorganization Committee, pp. 31–32.

11. *Op. cit.,* HEW Medicaid Recommendations, pp. 12–13.

12. *Ibid.* (See also Appendix II).

13. *Ibid.,* p. 155.

14. President's Task Force, *op. cit.*

15. Reorganization Committee, *op. cit.,* p. 32.

16. HEW Medicaid Recommendations, *op. cit.,* p. 7.

17. *Ibid.*

18. President's Task Force, *op. cit.*

19. Interview, Claire Townsend with the administrator of Sligo Gardens Nursing Home, Maryland, August 10, 1970.

20. Interview, Claire Townsend with Robert Mayne, Director of Intermediary Operations, Assistant Bureau of the Social Security Administration, August 12, 1970.

21. The Group for the Advancement of Psychiatry, *Toward A Public Policy on Mental Health Care of the Elderly,* Vol. VIII, no. 79, New York, November, 1970.

22. *Op. cit.,* President's Task Force, pp. 43–44.

23. *Ibid.,* p. 44.

24. *Op. cit.,* HEW Medicaid Recommendations, Introduction, p. 7.

25. *Ibid.,* Summary, pp. 2–3.

26. *Ibid.,* Summary, p. 6.

27. *Ibid.,* Summary, pp. 6–7.

28. H.R. 17550, Section 227(d)(4), p. 112.

29. *Developments in Aging, 1969,* Report of the Special Committee on Aging, U.S. Senate, February 16, 1970, p. 91.

30. *Ibid.,* pp. 91–92.

31. *Ibid.,* pp. 99–100.

32. *Ibid.,* pp. 100–101.

33. *Ibid.,* p. 400.

34. American Association of Retired Persons, National Retired Teachers Association Legislative Objectives for 1970.

35. *Op. cit.,* President's Task Force, p. 8.

36. *Op. cit.,* Group for the Advancement of Psychiatry, p. 46.

37. *Op. cit., Developments in Aging,* p. 41.

38. *Ibid.*

APPENDIX I: LETTERS

From Silver Spring, Maryland:

I would like to express my appreciation for the devoted care the nurses and aides gave my sister. They did all anyone could to make her as comfortable and happy as possible.

Their kindness to her and to me means more than words can tell.

From Adelphi, Maryland:

Enclosed is the payment for Miss L. I want to thank you for the care and tell you how satisfied [she is] with it. She seems content and never has a complaint.

To Claire Townsend:

My wonderful little mother died in an Oklahoma nursing home, after four and a half years of *existing* in five different homes. Due to lack of the necessary finances, I was unable to provide the care in my own home which she needed. She was bedfast, and I work. So, with state aid, we were able to keep her in these various nursing homes.

Each time we changed her from one to another, it was with the despairing hope that there would be an improvement in the conditions. There never was. She received *custodial* care if she was lucky. I visited her every day, so that she would know that I loved her, though giving her to strangers. She was lonely, frightened, bewildered, ill-cared for all those years. I still shudder at the thought of what she went through, and she deserved so very much more.

I had been impressed by the modern building we put her in at first. The grounds were well kept, the furniture was good. There seemed to be plenty of white uniforms. Then I learned that this was all a "front."

Catheters are inserted needed or not, so that the bedding can be left longer without changing. Also, catheters cut down on answering bells and lights for toilet needs. I regularly found the call light out of my mother's reach anyway. The staff found this cut down on duties. I observed this in other rooms also.

My mother was served meals without her dentures being put in. She was heaved up into a chair and left there until she fell on her face from exhaustion. Her food was cold and not cut up so she could eat it with her one good hand. I think those who are bedfast from strokes probably suffer most from inadequate care. She was roughly handled when her small fragile bones needed tenderness. An aide carelessly caught her arm in a bed rail one day resulting in a mass of black and blue bruises. She was left alone on the toilet one day, falling forward to suffer a head injury. Ambulatory patients came and went in her room at night, dazedly getting into bed with her and frightening her into seizures.

Frankly, I would rather kill myself than go through what she did.

And what can you do? I protested again and again, nothing changed in spite of assurances to the contrary.

Some aides care and some don't. All of them receive inadequate preliminary training. Too often they insert catheters, give shots, and handle patients without knowing what they are doing. Sometimes they lie about their experience because they need the jobs so badly.

I think inspection of nursing homes should be unannounced if possible, and at various times like morning or during late night hours.

It is too late to help my mother but the other poor old souls who live in the forgotten land of the nursing homes need your continuing efforts to help them.

Nursing homes are places to go and die, and rot away in the process.

No address given:

Words fail to express to you and your staff at the wonderful, kind, and sympathetic treatment given to my dear mother in her last days.

No one could have asked for more—not only the personal feelings you all had toward mother, but to us, the family.

I shall never forget and will always be deeply grateful for your extreme sincere kindness.

From Baltimore, Maryland:

We are writing this letter as an official record to state our high opinion of the professional and efficient way you operate the * * * nursing home. To each and every member of the staff, all employees, we want to extend our many thanks for the excellent care and attention given to our husband and father. For all the kind acts, constant supervision and understanding of Mr. P.'s long illness, we again say thanks from the bottom of our hearts.

Our feelings run very deep in this matter since Mr. P. was sick and confined to another home for several years. We spent many hours with him in this other institution and we can truly go on record that our experiences have been vast and heartbreaking. No attention was given to his physical or mental needs, and he was always left alone with his illness. These are our memories of this other so-called nursing home.

So to all patients, their families and friends we say be grateful every day that you have your beloved one in such a fine place as * * * nursing home, and please be as thankful as we are to all the dedicated people connected with its work of helping and taking care of the sick and incurable.

From Bay Harbor Islands, Florida:

I will be happy to give you any information you desire, from a personal and painful experience with several [nursing homes].

In several instances I had made my complaints to the Board of Health down here (Department of Nursing) and was advised that they would look into the matter. Nothing was done. I have one letter to testify that they had investigated and that condition would be corrected, but nothing changed.

They operate with a skeletal force of R.N.s; perhaps one for 150 or 200 patients. At night, according to law, they told me, they have only a licensed practical nurse, and a few aides, who, I found, had a very limited mental capacity and were almost sadistic in their treatment of these poor elderly at their mercy. I was a daily visitor when my mother was there and, therefore, saw and heard and was witness to more than the owners would have liked to have me see.

I know for a fact that my mother had been given injections in the night to keep her quiet because I found her completely sedated when I arrived the next noon, and this only because she needed attention and called for the nurse. [The situation] is inconceivable until you have had the personal experience, and I would be more than happy to assist you in any way possible.

To Congressman David Pryor:

There are sixty patients where I work and they are nearly all old and suffering, not so much from the cares which afflict their bodies but from the monotony and loneliness which living in a convalescent home implies.

I found this kind of suffering even penetrating the first nursing home I worked at, where the patients' physical care was more than adequate and where some attempt was made to involve them in social activities. But even there the staff was often inadequate for the number of patients. I soon came to realize though that the patient care at that particular rest home was the exception rather than the rule.

Having familiarized myself with the condition of the rest homes, I am horrified at the existing state of affairs.

As soon as one enters the sanitarium where I work, one is hit by the sense of meaninglessness in the lives of the patients. The hospital has one circular corridor and the patients that can, go around and around all day, their posey belts substituting for the chains of a supposedly more primitive time. I have known old ladies of eighty and some years to sit in the same wheel chairs from 9:00 in the morning until 8:00 at night without being taken to the bathroom; one lady had her buttocks covered with blisters from sitting so long.

I have seen patients who could walk when they came in, tied in wheelchairs because they are "nuisances" and then gradually lose all ability to walk because they have lost the use of their leg muscles.

I have been told to take care of the private patients first and the Medicare ones second, regardless of who needs the help the most. I have heard the head R.N. say to forget about washing the patient and just to put a clean top sheet on and tidy up the room so that everything will look good when visitors come.

I have asked myself why these conditions exist in a wealthy state such as California and in a wealthy nation. The patients pay $550 to $800 a month where I work, for a service that does not include medications or physician's fees; where the staff are paid $1.65 an hour with raises of ten cents after three months and a nickel after every following six months; where certain necessities such as powder, lotion, and tissues are to be bought by the patients and relatives. . . .

In regard to doctor care, the situation is also horrendous.

One doctor would come in on Sunday once in a while with his two small children to see his patients' charts and then leave. I used to think that he was paying them an extra visit, and I mentioned how nice it was that he found the time to inquire about his patients. The L.P.N. replied the visits on Sunday were the only ones he ever made and that all he did was look at the charts and leave, sending each patient a bill for forty dollars.

At the first hospital where I worked a man became critically ill and the R.N. called the doctor and asked him to come immediately. The doctor said he would be over in a few hours. Thinking he had misunderstood, she explained the situation, to which the doctor replied, "Look, he's old and he's got to go sometime." One lady who had passed away lay in her room for four hours until a doctor could be found to certify that she was dead. Then there was one lady whom I couldn't bathe because she needed a doctor's order and no one wanted to call him on Saturday. . . .

There are no social activities except travel films and a lady who comes to sing once in a while. Even the television is broken and nobody has bothered to fix it. The paint is peeling off the walls and the bathtubs are stained. Last Sunday I saw three cockroaches crawling up the wall and one in the packets of sugar. They say they come in with the food but I never saw any at the other place I worked. . . .

The old people wear rags pinned together if they have no caring relatives. They have on odd shoes and odd socks and whatever else we can find. I have taken clothes in only for them to be torn apart by the old washing machine and the harsh detergent.

The owner doesn't care. She said to one nurse that she had never learned anything about old people and didn't see why she should now; and if you didn't like it here you should go somewhere else, as if that was the point of it all.

I'm sick of the smell of urine and feces and the silent eyes of old people who have no one left; forced to die in a place that has no regard for their dignity or worth as human beings. The owners of these places are merchants of human flesh whose only concern is profit.

The patients have four walls to look at all day; and three meals and three doses of medication to quiet them down; and three shifts to note coming on and going off.

But one day is no different from the rest and even the sane patients don't know what day it is when you ask them, although some have calendars to mark off the days like the days off sentences to which they have been forced to serve. I have had patients ask me why God doesn't let them die and I have no answer.

There is a certain absurdity to the whole thing—these mainly rich old people left to decay and die in loneliness and rags. A woman with no one and nothing but a fortune in shares asked me of what use was all her money now. And the sad thing was it wasn't of any use except to pay her hospital bills.

Many times I felt that I could stand it no longer and that working for such people was only perpetuating the conditions. But someone has to do it. . . .

I am twenty-one and I could say it won't happen to me or those I love—but in the long run that doesn't matter. What is going on today is bad enough and we can't sweep our old people under the rug and pretend they don't exist. If we have the means to keep them alive we have the means to allow them to live a meaningful old age. . . .

From Connecticut:

My grandmother was sent from the * * * hospital in Putnam, Connecticut, to the * * * hospital in Willimantic, Connecticut, with a broken hip, and with the instructions that she should continue therapy and have her stitches removed. Instead we saw her condition get worse day by day. She was very incoherent, lost all interest in everything, got bedsores, lost a considerable amount of weight, and had no therapy at all.

We were very fortunate to find a vacancy at the * * * hospital in Manchester, Connecticut. Within twenty minutes after her arrival, her twenty-five-day-old stitches, with the flesh grown over them, were removed. She was given an air mattress for the bedsores, an overhead suspension bar to lift herself, a foot board to free her feet, and medication for severe urine burns. When told by the head nurse that they were glad to have her, it's no wonder she cried as she answered, "I'm glad to be here." On the third day she was dressed and outside in a wheelchair for fresh air. We are now waiting for a report from the hospital so they can start her daily therapy.

It's such a blessing to find dedicated people who care and to see all the good they are doing and not to hear old people crying continually for help only to be ignored.

A full investigation should be conducted to stop these hospitals from filling their patients full of pills, putting their buzzers out of their reach, and not bringing any food at all, only because they can't be bothered.

Seeing all the cruelty that takes place in this sort of convalescent hospital doesn't give a person much incentive to want to reach the "golden years" of their life. . . .

From Oregon:

I have read you are making an investigation of conditions

in nursing homes. I have been a patient for some time following amputation of both legs. I am also deaf, but things I have seen and experienced convinced me I should write. . . .

I have seen nurses aides tease these old people to make them mad, just for sport. The patients rebel and try to fight back but can do little to defend themselves but yell and throw food from bed or wheelchairs.

One woman was here temporarily until she could be transferred to a mental hospital in Salem. She screamed at night and was moved to an isolated room so she wouldn't disturb other patients. A couple days later I asked about her and she was dead. There was nothing evidently wrong with her otherwise—I've never heard of insanity alone being fatal?

The bone in my leg is exposed and draining. The dressings are never changed oftener than once a week and as infrequently as two and a half weeks.

June 22: I had a shampoo—the first this year—then only because I complained.

Visitors tell me that sometimes walking in here is like visiting a zoo—the odor. . . .

Something must be done for those patients unable to help themselves and who have no family to see they are cared for—I feel it would be more humane to put them to sleep than to neglect, starve, and abuse them.

Most of the staff here are wonderful, but just a few indifferent and snotty aides cause so much unhappiness. These people for the most part have been rejected by their families, are lonely, and ill—old age is so undignified. . . .

From Illinois:

My son was an invalid and died at the age of twenty-one —last October—after having spent five years in nursing homes. He was blind and immobile and could not stand or feed himself. My husband is a mental patient. . . . In spite of the hardship, as I have another son to care for, I drove every day to see and care for my son—as the care was so poor in all nursing homes he was in. . . . Thousands and thousands of dollars must have been spent by the state for his care—and I feel he received none.

His death certificate speaks for itself. He contracted a flu virus last fall, and because he had received no care and only improper feeding, he died. I was threatened and abused every day—because I asked why.

Four months before he died, I received a letter from the * * * nursing home. He was to be removed immediately. When I asked why, I was told I broke all the rules—by feeding him between meals. . . . I never fed him after that because I was afraid—and the death certificate tells the rest.

. . . [Immediate cause: pneumonia, terminal; other significant conditions: malnutrition, severe, due to inadequate food
intake.]

From California:

On night shifts, changing of soiled linens is done by re-
placing soiled with fresh, clean linen. Sheets wet with urine
are thrown over back staircases, stairwells, etc., to dry. Then
used to replace freshly wetted sheets under the next incontinent patient when sheets are "changed." The stench is
startling. . . .

No address given:

This world would be a much better place if there had
never been a nursing home. . . . There's thousands of
active old ladies on Social Security or pension who cannot
afford a place alone—who would be thankful for an opportunity to care for the disabled for free home and little pay.

APPENDIX II: SUMMARY OF PERTINENT LAWS

Health Insurance for the Aged—Hospital Insurance: (Also known as Medicare, Title XVIII, Part A of the Social Security Act.)*

Purpose: This program provides hospital insurance protection for covered services to any person sixty-five or over who is entitled to Federally administered Social Security or railroad retirement benefits (although workers, their spouses, and widows can qualify for monthly benefits under various options before age sixty-five). A dependent spouse or survivor sixty-five or over is entitled to Medicare based on the worker's record. The covered protection in each benefit period includes hospital inpatient care; posthospital extended care; and home health visits by nurses or other health workers from a participating home health agency. It does not include doctors' services or drugs.

Funding: Under Social Security, workers, their employers, and self-employed people pay a contribution based on earnings during their working years. At sixty-five, the portion of their contribution that has gone into a special Hospital In-

---

* This summary of the Medicare program is taken from an article published by the Group for the Advancement of Psychiatry: *Toward A Public Policy on Mental Health Care of the Elderly,* Vol. III, no. 79, New York, November, 1970.

All other program summaries, except as otherwise indicated, are taken directly from a Report of the Committee on Government Operations of the United States Senate, Subcommittee on Executive Reorganization and Government Research, entitled a *Federal Role in Health,* published April 30, 1970, pp. 67–125.

surance Trust Fund guarantees that workers will have help in paying hospital bills.

Financial Data: The total contributions paid in fiscal 1970 were $4,758,000,000.

Responsibility: Social Security Administration, U.S. Department of Health, Education and Welfare.

Health Insurance for the Aged—Supplementary Medical Insurance: (Also known as Medicare, Title XVIII, Part B of the Social Security Act.)

Social Security's Supplementary Medical Insurance program is voluntary, and no one is covered automatically. Medical Insurance helps pay for many of the costs of illness not covered by Hospital Insurance—doctors' bills, outpatient hospital services, medical supplies and services, home health services, outpatient physical therapy, and other health care services.

Eligibility: Protection is offered to those sixty-five and over if they sign up for it within a specified period—within three years after their first opportunity (e.g., when they reach age sixty-five or qualify under various options before they reach sixty-five). Participants must also pay monthly premiums.

Funding: Supplementary Medical Insurance is not financed through payroll deductions and is not based on earnings or period of work. Monthly premiums are required of each enrollee; these premiums are backed by the same amount from the Federal government which pays its half through general revenue. Monthly premiums for fiscal 1971 are $5.30. The premium may be changed for fiscal 1972 by announcement of the Secretary of Health, Education and Welfare before December 31, 1970.

Financial Data: Premiums paid for fiscal 1970 amounted to $922 million. Federal contributions were $928 million. Payments totalled $1,949,000,000.

Responsibility: Social Security Administration, U.S. Department of Health, Education and Welfare.

Medical Assistance Program: (Also known as Medicaid, Title XIX of the Social Security Act.)*

Purpose: This program provides grants to states to administer medical assistance programs for low-income persons.

Eligibility: (1) the needy—all public assistance recipients in the Federally aided categories (the aged, blind, disabled,

---

* Summary taken from an article published by the Group for the Advancement of Psychiatry: *Toward A Public Policy on Mental Health Care of the Elderly,* Vol. III, no. 79, New York, November, 1970.

and families with dependent children) and those who would qualify for that assistance under Federal regulations; (2) at a state's option, the medically needy—people in the four groups mentioned above who have enough income or resources for daily needs but not for medical expenses; and (3) all children under twenty-one whose parents cannot afford medical care.

Funding: Expenditures are shared by Federal and state governments, according to the various states' per capita income.

Financial Data: Medicaid cost the Federal government $4.8 billion in fiscal 1970, or about 52 per cent of the total cost of the program. The program paid medical bills for some thirteen million people.

Responsibility: Social and Rehabilitation Service of the U.S. Department of Health, Education and Welfare.

Old Age Assistance—Maintenance Payments:

Purpose: This is a public assistance program providing financial help to states to make income-maintenance payments to poor people who are age sixty-five or over. All states have Old Age Assistance programs.

Eligibility: A needy aged person applies for Old Age Assistance to the local welfare agency. To be eligible, he must be at least sixty-five years old. He must also meet his state's eligibility requirements pertaining to income.

Financial Data: OAA payments paid by the Federal government totaled $1,336,071,000 in fiscal 1970. Of this amount, some $163,702,000 went to Intermediate Care Facilities. More than 50 per cent of the program is paid by Federal funds. As of April, 1970, some 2,050,000 persons were registered.

Responsibility: Assistance Payments Administration, Social and Rehabilitation Service, U.S. Department of Health, Education and Welfare, and state and local welfare agencies.

Foster Grandparent Program:

Purpose: To give emotionally deprived children needed affection and attention, and to provide new roles and functions for older people with low incomes, enabling them to maintain a sense of dignity and usefulness, as well as demonstrating a major resource of responsible workers for communities and social agencies.

Eligibility: Applicant group may be any public or nonprofit private organization or institution.

Funding: The Foster Grandparent Program is funded by the Office of Economic Opportunity through its Community Action Program.

Financial Data: $8.9 million was spent in fiscal 1970 to

fund sixty-eight programs in forty states and Puerto Rico. Twenty per cent matching funds are required. No new programs have been funded since 1968.

Responsibility: The Administration on Aging of the Social and Rehabilitation Service of the U.S. Department of Health, Education and Welfare.

Community Planning and Services:

Purpose: Title III of the Older American Act provides for allotment of funds to states to strengthen state agencies on aging and to enable states to make grants to local public and private nonprofit agencies providing services to older people, for community planning and coordination of programs, for demonstration programs, and for training of special personnel.

Eligibility: Allotments are paid to states with approved state plans and a single state agency for administering the plan.

Funding: One per cent of the annual appropriation is available for each state. The remainder is appropriated according to the ratio of the state's population aged sixty-five years and older to the total population aged sixty-five and older. Unused allotments are reallocated. Federal funds may cover 75 per cent of cost per project for the first year, 60 per cent the second, and 50 per cent the third. Support terminates after the third year, and continuation must be provided for by the state or private funding.

Financial data: $9 million was appropriated in fiscal 1970.

Responsibility: The Office of State and Community Services of the Administration on Aging, Social and Rehabilitation Service, U.S. Department of Health, Education and Welfare.

Hospital and Medical Facilities Construction—The Hill-Burton Program:

Purpose: This is a program of grants and loans for construction, modernization, or replacement of diagnostic or treatment centers, hospitals for chronically ill, rehabilitation facilities, nursing homes, hospitals, public health centers, in accordance with a mandatory state plan revised annually.

Eligibility: States are awarded appropriations on a population-based formula, weighted for financial ability and need. Private nonprofit organizations, states, and other public agencies may receive grants or loans.

Financial Data: A matching rate is established by the states each year, between 33⅓ per cent and 66⅔ per cent by statutory limits. $172.2 million was authorized for fiscal year 1970—$27.1 million for modernization; $54.2 million for hospital public health centers; $63.6 for long term care facilities; $18.2 million for diagnostic and treatment centers; and $9.1 million for rehabilitation facilities. This was a decrease of some $8 million from fiscal 1969.

Responsibility: The Health Facilities Planning and Construction Service, Public Health Service, U.S. Department of Health, Education and Welfare, and the state agencies administering the Hill-Burton program.

Elderly and Handicapped—Housing Mortgage Insurance:

Purpose: To help meet the housing needs of elderly people and of handicapped people, the National Housing Act authorizes the Federal Housing Administration to insure mortgages for financing rental housing projects designed specifically for occupants age sixty-two and older, or for the handicapped of any age. Projects may be new or rehabilitated, with eight or more dwelling units.

Eligibility: Both nonprofit and profit-motivated sponsors are eligible. The sponsors may be either private individuals, corporations, associations, or trusts.

Financial Data: The Federal Housing Administration insures loans made by approved lending institutions. Maximum amount the FHA insures is $12.5 million. The maximum interest rate is 6¾ per cent. The maximum term is forty years. The insurance is up to 100 per cent of the cost for nonprofit, and up to 90 per cent for profit-motivated sponsors.

The direct loan program virtually came to an end in fiscal 1970, with no funds made available for this purpose. Under section 236 of the Act, some $16 million was made available for interest subsidies, totaling $284 million of insured mortgages.

Responsibility: The local Federal Housing Insuring Office and the Assistance Commissioner for Subsidized Housing Programs, U.S. Department of Housing and Urban Development.

Nursing Home Mortgage Insurance:

Purpose: To help provide needed nursing homes, adequate in safety and proper care of occupants. The Federal Housing Administration insures mortgages both for building new nursing homes and for rehabilitating existing ones. At least twenty beds in the nursing home are necessary for participation in this mortgage insurance.

Eligibility: A corporation, a trust, a partnership, or an individual may be a proprietary mortgager. A nonprofit mortgager may be a private corporation or association, organized for purposes other than making profit for itself or persons identified with it.

Financial Data: The maximum mortgage the insurance

will cover is $12.5 million per project. The highest insured amount is 90 per cent of the Federal Housing Administration's estimated value of the completed project and equipment. The term of coverage can be for no more than twenty years. The maximum permissible interest rate is 6¾ per cent.

In 1969, there were ninety insured projects for amounts totaling $93,601,200 and involving 10,888 beds. That same year, there were 128 applications involving a total of $127,-534,587 and 15,009 beds.

Responsibility: The local Federal Housing Administration Insuring Office and the Elderly, Nursing Homes and Medical Facilities Branch of the U.S. Department of Housing and Urban Development.

Manpower Development and Training Act:

Purpose: To train and retrain unemployed and underemployed, dealing with problems of obsolete skills, jobless, need for basic education; to reclaim hard-core unemployed; to focus on need for trained personnel in skill shortage categories.

Eligibility: Public or private agencies, community organizations, governments, trade or industrial associations, labor organizations. Also individual employers may receive contracts for training programs.

Funding: Funds are provided for occupations training (institutional, on-the-job, basic education, special programs for the disadvantaged, ages sixteen to twenty-one; workers forty-five years and older). Full Federal financing is provided in specific redevelopment areas—research, experimental, and demonstration projects; placement.

Financial Data: Training institutions are paid 90 per cent of training costs; state pays 10 per cent. Matching may be in kind or in cash. Employers or other sponsors provide training facilities and pay trainee wages for hours spent in production of goods and services entering interstate commerce.

Responsibility: The Local State Employment Service or Regional Office, or the Bureau of Work Training Programs is the U.S. Department of Labor.

Comprehensive Health Centers:

Purpose: In poverty areas where health services are seriously lacking, grants are provided for establishment of Comprehensive Health Centers offering treatment, preventive health services, rehabilitation, dental care, family planning, and mental health services. Also drugs and appliances, personal and community health education, social services, and other health centers must be integrated or coordinated with existing publicly supported health services in the area.

Eligibility: Public and private nonprofit organizations such as medical schools, medical societies, hospitals, clinics, group practice plans, and public health departments may be operating agencies.

Financial Data: $90 million was appropriated for fiscal year 1969.

Responsibility: Local Community Action agencies or the Regional Office of the Office of Economic Opportunity.

Health Care Programs of the Veteran's Administration:

The Veteran's Administration offers several programs of assistance to veterans needing health care: hospitalization, with first priority to disabilities or diseases incurred or aggravated in military service; skilled nursing home care following hospitalization or for domiciliary residents; domiciliary care for disabled veterans, nursing home care in veteran's community; assistance to eligible blind veterans for rehabilitation; prostheses for service-connected disabilities.

Eligibility: May be determined in individual cases. States furnishing such care and assistance are also eligible to apply for financial assistance.

Responsibility: A Veteran's Service Organization representative or a Veteran's Administration Hospital or a Veteran's Administration Regional Office.

APPENDIX III

QUESTIONS TO ASK WHEN VISITING A NURSING HOME

1. Does the home offer progressive stages of care, or at least the one you're interested in?
   Residential care: provides room and board, help with laundry, shopping, and cleaning;
   Personal care: provides help with walking, bathing, getting dressed, and eating; preparation of special diets;
   Nursing care: provides professional medical care, involving the administering of medication, the insertion of catheters, injections—all at doctor's orders.
2. Is the home licensed by the state? (This is a legal requirement; unfortunately, it is not an indication of reliability.)
3. Is the home certified for Medicare and Medicaid? (If not, the home is not receiving any Federal funds.)
4. What is the cost of the home? Is everything covered by the monthly rate, or are there a lot of "extras" tacked on?
5. When was the last inspection made? When was the last Federal inspection made? How often is the facility inspected?
6. Does the home require a complete physical before entrance, or immediately upon arrival? Is there also a questionnaire to be filled out dealing with the patient's hobbies, favorite pastimes, etc.?
7. If the patient's personal physician will not continue care after entrance into the home, does the home require a written transferral from that doctor to one of the doctors in the home?

8. Does the home have emergency admission arrangements with one or more of the general hospitals in the area?

9. Does the home have regular dental services? Are they "extra"?

10. Who is the owner of the home? Is there a conflict of interest, i.e., is he a doctor, pharmacist, or does he have an interest in profit-making concerns related to the ·home?

11. Does the owner require entrance contracts that fail to promise a return of property if a patient leaves the home? (Always get an entrance contract checked by a lawyer.)

12. What are the qualifications of the administrator?

13. How large is the nursing staff?

14. Is there a registered nurse on duty full-time?

15. Are the licensed practical nurses graduates of approved schools of practical nursing?

16. How large is the staff—including nurses, doctors, kitchen help, laundry help, maintenance men, etc.? (One staff member to every three beds is the national average. Federal standards raise the ratio.)

17. How many patients are bedridden? (If large numbers are confined to their beds, it might indicate a lack of staff.)

18. Is there an in-service training program for the nurse's aides? (This shows a willingness on the part of the home to improve the quality of care.)

19. Is there a good rapport between the staff and the patients?

20. Are the patients clean? Is their hair neat, clean, and combed? Are their finger- and toenails clean and cut? Is there an extra charge for washing hair or for cutting nails?

21. Are the bedrooms neat and clean?

22. Are the emergency buzzers within reach of the patients? Do the nurses respond to these calls quickly?

23. Is there any urine smell in the home? Or a heavy cover-up smell?

24. Does the home have a regular dietician? (Ask to see the kitchen.)

25. Is the menu posted and followed? Are there different diets for patients who require them?

26. Does the staff eat the same food as the residents?

27. How many residents use the dining room? Do they seem to enjoy their meals?

28. Is the food served attractively?

29. Do the bedridden patients receive hot food?

30. At what hours are the meals served? (Some homes serve all the meals within one shift to save money.)

31. Does the home charge extra for hand feeding? (This is ridiculous, since the need for being fed may well be the reason for institutionalization in the first place.)

32. Is the facility pleasing in appearance?

33. Are there paintings and decorations on the walls?

34. Are the surroundings cold, impersonal, hard to adjust to?

35. Is the home situated in the country? (It may be more beautiful and less expensive than in the city, but there may also be less community involvement, no public transportation, and few visitors.)

36. Is there a sprinkler system and fire extinguishers? Is there a heat and smoke sensor system, with an automatic direct alarm line hooked up with the local fire station?

37. Are there handrails along the halls? Guardrails in the bathrooms?

38. Do the patients use the living rooms? Are they merely for appearance, or for use by the staff?

39. Does the home provide occupational therapy? Physical therapy? Recreational therapy?

40. Is there a therapist who works often enough to fulfill the patients' needs?

41. Is the therapy room large and well equipped?

42. Does the institution provide a physical therapist to teach the patients to use the toilet and other facilities in their own rooms?

43. Are there books, magazines, and television provided for entertainment? Are they the only entertainment? (Ask to see the list of activities for that month.)

44. Are visitors encouraged to come? (If visiting hours are restricted at all, perhaps the nursing home is trying to hide something.)

45. Do the patients seem happy? Would *you* feel happy leaving your mother there?

APPENDIX IV: PEOPLE TO CONTACT

DEPARTMENT OF HEALTH, EDUCATION, AND WELFARE

Regional Offices and Directors

REGION I—BOSTON, MASSACHUSETTS (Connecticut, Massachusetts, Maine, New Hampshire, Vermont, Rhode Island)
Harold Putnam (617) 223-6831
John Fitzgerald Kennedy Building
Government Center
Boston, Massachusetts 02203

REGION II—NEW YORK, NEW YORK (New York, New Jersey, Puerto Rico, Virgin Islands)
Bernice L. Bernstein (212) 264-4600
Federal Building
26 Federal Plaza
New York, New York 10007

REGION III—PHILADELPHIA, PENNSYLVANIA (Delaware, District of Columbia, Maryland, Pennsylvania, Virginia, West Virginia)
Bernard V. McCusty (703) 296-1221 or (215) 597-9050
401 North Broad Street
Philadelphia, Pennsylvania 19108

REGION IV—ATLANTA, GEORGIA (Alabama, Florida, Georgia, Kentucky, Mississippi, North Carolina, South Carolina, Tennessee)
Cary H. Hall (404) 526-5817
Peachtree–Seventh Building
50–7th Street, N.E. Room 404
Atlanta, Georgia 30323

REGION V—CHICAGO, ILLINOIS (Illinois, Indiana, Minnesota, Michigan, Ohio, Wisconsin)
  Harold Boath (312) 353-5160
  New Post Office Building, Room 712
  433 West Van Buren Street
  Chicago, Illinois 60607

REGION VI—DALLAS, TEXAS (Missouri, Iowa, Kansas, Nebraska)
  Charles C. Green (214) 749-3396
  1114 Commerce Street
  Dallas, Texas 75202

REGION VII—KANSAS CITY, MISSOURI (Arkansas, Louisiana, New Mexico, Oklahoma, Texas)
  Max Milo Mills (816) 374-3436
  Federal Office Building
  601 East 12th Street
  Kansas City, Missouri 64106

REGION VIII—DENVER, COLORADO (Colorado, Montana, North Dakota, South Dakota, Utah, Wyoming)
  William T. Van Orman (303) 297-3373
  Federal Office Building, Room 9017
  19th and Stout Streets
  Denver, Colorado 80202

REGION IX—SAN FRANCISCO, CALIFORNIA (Arizona, California, Hawaii, Guam, Wake Island, American Samoa, Trust Territories of the Pacific Islands)
  Robert T. Coop (415) 556-6746
  Federal Office Building
  50 Fulton Street
  San Francisco, California 94102

REGION X—SEATTLE, WASHINGTON (Alaska, Idaho, Oregon, Washington)
  Bernard E. Kelley (206) 583-4304
  Arcade Building
  1319 Second Avenue
  Seattle, Washington

DEPARTMENT OF HEALTH, EDUCATION AND WELFARE
  330 Independence Avenue, S.W.
  Washington, D.C. 20201 (202) 963-1110
  Secretary Elliott Richardson
    Room 5246–HEW (202) 962-2351
  Undersecretary John Veneman
    Room 5262–HEW (202) 963-6156

Public Health Service

Parklawn Building
5600 Fishers Lane
Rockville, Maryland 20852

Acting Chief of Nursing Home Branch
Dr. Paul Pedersen
Room 7A 55 (301) 443-1450

Home Health Branch
Acting Chief
Harold Dame
Room 7A 30 (301) 443-1390

Social and Rehabilitation Service

Administration on Aging
Commissioner John Martin
Room 3086–HEW (202) 963-3581

Chief, Reports and Analysis Section
Herman Brotman
Room 3614–HEW (202) 963-6713

Medical Services Administration (Medicaid)
Commissioner Howard Newman
Room 4094–HEW (202) 963-4958

Assistant to the Commissioner
Frank Frantz
Room 4086–HEW (202) 962-1259

Rehabilitation Services Administration
Commissioner Edward Newman
Room 3006–HEW (202) 962-2335

Social Security Administration

6401 Security Boulevard
Baltimore, Maryland 21235 (301) 944-5000

Commissioner Robert Ball
Room 900 SS (301) 944-5000

Deputy Commissioner
Arthur Hess
Room 900 SS (301) 944-5000

Assistant to the Commissioner
Hugh Johnson
Room 900 SS (301) 944-5000

Press Officer
Charlotte Crenson

Room 103 SS (301) 944-5000

SSA Bureau of Health Insurance (Medicare)
Director
Thomas Tierney
Room 700 SS (301) 944-5000 Ext. 2971

Assistant to Director
David Kopelman
Room 700 SS (301) 944-5000

Division of Intermediary Operations
Director Robert Mayne
Room 4R12 SS (301) 944-5000

Division of State Operations

Director
Morris Levy
Room 4F1 SS (301) 944-5000

Deputy Director
Gerald Sheinback *
Room 4G1 SS (301) 944-5000

American Nursing Home Association

1025 Connecticut Avenue, N.W.
Suite 607
Washington, D.C. 20036 (202) 833-2050

American Association of Homes for the Aging

National Press Building
529–14th Street, N.W.
Washington, D.C. 20004 (202) 347-2000

National Council of Health Care Services

Berkeley Bennett or
Elizabeth Connell
1625 I Street, N.W.
Washington, D.C. 20006 (202) 659-8255

American Association of Retired Persons

Mrs. Lara Buckingham
1225 Connecticut Avenue, N.W.
Washington, D.C. 20036 (202) 659-4670

---

* Sheinback would like to receive complaint letters in order to take appropriate action.

National Council of Senior Citizens
William Hutton, Executive Director
1627 K Street, N.W.
Washington, D.C. 20006 (202) 783-6850

Special Committee on Aging (Senate) (202) 225-5364
Chairman Frank Church (Idaho)
Harrison Williams (New Jersey)
Alan Bible (Nevada)
Jennings Randolph (West Virginia)
Edmund Muskie (Maine)
Frank Moss (Utah)
Edward Kennedy (Massachusetts)
Walter Mondale (Minnesota)
Vance Hartke (Indiana)
Claiborne Pell (Rhode Island)
Thomas Eagleton (Missouri)
Winston Prouty (Vermont)
Hiram Fong (Hawaii)
Jack Miller (Iowa)
Clifford Hansen (Wyoming)
Paul Fanin (Arizona)
Edward Gurney (Florida)
William Saxbe (Ohio)
(Two Republicans yet unnamed)

Subcommittee on Long-Term Care
Chairman Frank Moss

Val Halamanderas, Staff Director
Room G225 New Senate Office Building
Constitution Avenue
Washington, D.C. 20510 (202) 225-5364

CONGRESSMAN DAVID PRYOR (D.–ARK.)
307 Cannon House Office Building
Washington, D.C. 20515 (202) 225-3772

MOTHER MARY BERNADETTE DE LOURDES
St. Joseph's Manor
Trumbull, Connecticut 06611 (203) 268-6204

DR. ROBERT BUTLER
3815 Huntington Street, N.W.
Washington, D.C. 20015 (202) 966-4121

PRESIDENT RICHARD M. NIXON
The White House
Washington, D.C. 20500 (202) 456-1414

MAL SCHECHTOR, Washington editor of *Hospital Practice*
1230 National Press Building
Washington, D.C. 20004 (202) 628-7837

THEODORE SCHUCHAT, author of "Joys and Jolts of Retirement"
North American Newspaper Alliance
209 National Press Building
Washington, D.C. 20004 (202) 347-0141

APPENDIX V: BUREAUCRATIC FRAGMENTATION OF RESPONSIBILITY FOR NURSING HOMES

(*next page*)

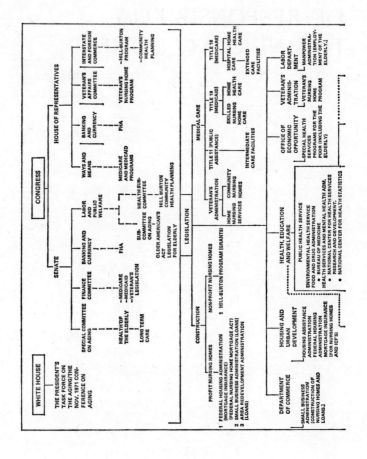

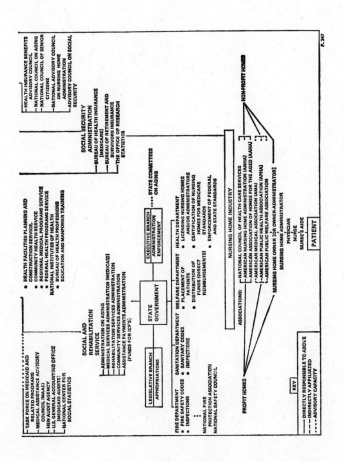

INDEX